CHALLENGING CHOICES

MCGILL-QUEEN'S/ASSOCIATED MEDICAL SERVICES
STUDIES IN THE HISTORY OF MEDICINE, HEALTH,
AND SOCIETY

Series editors: J.T.H. Connor and Erika Dyck

This series presents books in the history of medicine, health studies, and social policy, exploring interactions between the institutions, ideas, and practices of medicine and those of society as a whole. To begin to understand these complex relationships and their history is a vital step to ensuring the protection of a fundamental human right: the right to health. Volumes in this series have received financial support to assist publication from Associated Medical Services, Inc. (AMS), a Canadian charitable organization with an impressive history as a catalyst for change in Canadian healthcare. For eighty years, AMS has had a profound impact through its support of the history of medicine and the education of healthcare professionals, and by making strategic investments to address critical issues in our healthcare system. AMS has funded eight chairs in the history of medicine across Canada, is a primary sponsor of many of the country's history of medicine and nursing organizations, and offers fellowships and grants through the AMS History of Medicine and Healthcare Program (www.amshealthcare.ca).

Challenging Choices

*Canada's Population
Control in the 1970s*

ERIKA DYCK and MAUREEN LUX

McGill-Queen's University Press
Montreal & Kingston • London • Chicago

© McGill-Queen's University Press 2020

ISBN 978-0-2280-0374-8 (cloth)
ISBN 978-0-2280-0375-5 (paper)
ISBN 978-0-2280-0441-7 (ePDF)
ISBN 978-0-2280-0442-4 (ePUB)

Legal deposit fourth quarter 2020
Bibliothèque nationale du Québec

Printed in Canada on acid-free paper that is 100% ancient forest free
(100% post-consumer recycled), processed chlorine free

This book has been published with the help of a grant from the Canadian
Federation for the Humanities and Social Sciences, through the Awards to
Scholarly Publications Program, using funds provided by the Social Sciences
and Humanities Research Council of Canada.

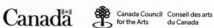

We acknowledge the support of the Canada Council for the Arts.

Nous remercions le Conseil des arts du Canada de son soutien.

Library and Archives Canada Cataloguing in Publication

Title: Challenging choices: Canada's population control in the 1970s /
Erika Dyck and Maureen Lux.

Names: Dyck, Erika, author. | Lux, Maureen K. (Maureen Katherine), author.

Series: McGill-Queen's/Associated Medical Services studies in the history
of medicine, health, and society; 54.

Description: Series statement: McGill-Queen's / Associated Medical Services
studies in the history of medicine, health, and society; 54 | Includes
bibliographical references and index.

Identifiers: Canadiana (print) 20200288687 | Canadiana (ebook) 20200288849 |
ISBN 9780228003748 (cloth) | ISBN 9780228003755 (paper) | ISBN
9780228004417 (ePDF) | ISBN 9780228004424 (ePUB)

Subjects: LCSH: Birth control—Social aspects—Canada—History—20th century—
Case studies. | LCSH: Birth control—Political aspects—Canada—History—
20th century—Case studies. | LCSH: Reproductive rights—Social aspects—
Canada—History—20th century—Case studies. | LCSH: Reproductive rights—
Political aspects—Canada—History—20th century—Case studies. | LCSH:
Reproductive health—Social aspects—Canada—History—20th century—Case
studies. | LCSH: Reproductive health—Political aspects—Canada—History—
20th century—Case studies. | LCGFT: Case studies.

Classification: LCC HQ766.5.C3 D93 2020 | DDC 363.9/6097109047—dc23

This book was typeset by Marquis Interscript in 10.5/13 Sabon.

Contents

Acknowledgments

Writing historical monographs can often be a lonely pursuit, but this project was ideally suited for a collaborative adventure. Working together on this book allowed us to bring different perspectives into the discussion, and although it sometimes created confusion, we ultimately believe that the product is richer for confronting some of the inherent contradictions and complexities that come from studying birth control and the ideas of choice that have politicized this subject over time.

We reached out to archival collections across the country and are grateful to the many research assistants who helped retrieve materials from archives far from our homes and teaching duties. Special thanks to Brent Brenyo, Matt DeCloedt, Leslie Digdon, Matthew Ginther, Adam Montgomery, Karissa Patton, Fedir Razumenko, Erin Spinney, Sarah Taggart, and Keegan Young. Thanks especially to Patrick Farrell, who read the entire manuscript and offered detailed feedback. We are also grateful to the many people who heard us present parts of the research along the way and whose comments and questions helped us refine and rethink our approaches to this topic. We presented some of these ideas at the 3 Societies meeting in Edmonton (Canadian History & Philosophy of Science, British History of Science, and American History of Science); the Social History of Medicine meeting in Canterbury; the centennial event celebrating women's suffrage organized by Sarah Carter and Nanci Langford in Edmonton; invited lectures to the Department of Sociology in Brno, Czech Republic; the Frie Institute in Berlin; the European History of Medicine meeting in Bucharest; and the University of Strathclyde's annual Centre for the Study of Health and Healthcare symposium in Glasgow. The scholarly feedback and exposure have helped us to locate our study of Canada within a broader set of discussions about birth control, feminism, and reproductive health activism.

We were very pleased to publish earlier versions of this work, which also helped to generate discussion about the project. Chapter 2 was published as "Population Control in the 'Global North'? Canada's Response to Aboriginal Reproductive Rights and Neo-Eugenics" in *Canadian Historical Review* 97, no. 4 (December 2016). Parts of chapter 3 were published in a previous form in *Preventing Mental Illness: Past, Present, and Future*, edited by Despo Kritsotaki, Vicky Long, and Matthew Smith (Palgrave Macmillan, 2018). We also shared some of the major findings from our work in a Conversation Canada article published in 2018.

The review process helped to refine some of our interpretations, for which we are grateful to the two anonymous peer reviewers and especially to Kyla Madden at MQUP, who expertly shepherded our manuscript through this process and answered all our many questions along the way.

This research received financial support from Canadian Institutes of Health Research (CIHR).

We acknowledge that with settler privileges come choices about families that many people in this book did not have. It is with humility that we tell their stories. We are also humbled by the people who have shared their painful stories of having their children or their ovaries taken away from them against their choices. We hope that writing this book helps to honour some of the many choices and different power dynamics that have shaped Canadian families.

Erika thanks her family and friends who have listened patiently and supported the late nights or extended travel to archives or conferences.

Maureen thanks her family for their constant support. Family comes in all sizes; it grows with wonder and joy, and shrinks with profound sadness and pain.

CHALLENGING CHOICES

Introduction

Many westerners by the mid-twentieth century would have been familiar with the dystopic writings of British author Aldous Huxley. His popular novel, *Brave New World*, published in 1932, introduced readers to a futuristic place where human reproduction was fiercely controlled and managed scientifically, fusing biology with governance in a dark and foreboding tale where over-organization (Huxley's expression for totalitarian management) meets overpopulation.[1] Huxley was also deeply connected to a legacy of British evolutionary biologists, his grandfather Thomas Huxley having been closely associated with Charles Darwin, and his brother, Julian Huxley, the head of the British Eugenics Society. Aldous was always enchanted by the intersections of science and society, and in *Brave New World* he explored how overpopulation, coupled with a growing modern desire to control, would evolve into a more natural form of tyranny that eroded democratic institutions. In *Brave New World* Huxley even fantasizes about a fictitious pill (before the creation of the actual birth control pill), and he foreshadows the ethical dilemma facing modern civilization. He suggests in his 1958 *Brave New World Revisited* that

we are given two choices – famine, pestilence, and war on the one hand, birth control on the other. Most of us choose birth control – and immediately find ourselves confronted by a problem that is simultaneously a puzzle in physiology, pharmacology, sociology, psychology and even theology. "The Pill" has not yet been invented. When and if it is invented, how can it be distributed to the many hundreds of millions of potential mothers (or, if it is a pill that works upon the male, potential fathers) who will have to take it if the birth rate of the species is to be reduced? And, given existing social customs and the forces of cultural and psychological inertia, how can those who ought to take the pill, but don't want to, be persuaded to change their minds? And what about the objections on the part of the Roman Catholic Church, to any form of birth control except the so-called Rhythm Method – a method, incidentally, which has proved, hitherto, to be almost completely ineffective in reducing the birth rate of those industrially backward societies where such a reduction is most urgently necessary? And these questions about the future, hypothetical Pill must be asked, with as little prospect of eliciting satisfactory answers, about the chemical and mechanical methods of birth control already available.[2]

Huxley's novel played with the concept of a birth control pill whose mechanical use was somewhat simple, but the moral and ethical considerations surrounding its consumption were murky, even contradictory at times. Huxley titillated readers with these ideas only a few years before G.D. Searle introduced the first generation of birth control pills.

By the time Huxley revisited his brave new world concept in 1958, birth control as a concept, and *the* birth control pill, as a specific device, had gathered new momentum in the public imagination. Contraception was not itself new, but the introduction of the birth control pill changed the tenor of debates about family planning and population control by introducing new contraceptive technologies with far-ranging possibilities for distribution.[3] Huxley's further musings on this issue may have prepared readers for some of the larger moral tensions that surrounded the introduction of the Pill, as a simple, discrete, and potentially affordable and packaged response to a much larger set of political, economic, and moral conversations about population control. Huxley's fictitious pill attuned readers to the global ramifications of birth control and the need to recognize how this tiny pill had far-reaching consequences for gender relations, economics, and governance.

The Pill became a reality in 1961, and Huxley's predictions came true. Population control had reemerged as a critical issue by the end of the decade, prompting global leaders to take stock of the uneven distribution of resources and people around the world. Solutions to the so-called fertility burden required careful multilateral management by states and moral guidance by religious and political leaders on the world stage. Most of the attention to population growth focused primarily on the Global South, where claims of overcrowding, poverty, and disease helped to resurrect ideas about the consequences of evolutionary biology coupled with the relative lack of sufficient resources, linking concerns about the environment and human welfare. The birth control pill offered a technological solution and became a symbol of hope for stemming the tide of overpopulation, at least in theory.

By the time the birth control pill was a reality, the moral terrain about which Huxley had philosophized was indeed complicated, and many of the official suggestions from policy makers as to who should embrace the Pill were at odds with the history of who had lobbied for access to birth control for personal use. Taking or rejecting the birth control pill implied different political views on reproduction and choice. Throughout the 1970s in Canada this conversation became rife with contradictions as to how using contraception might appreciably contribute to the national economy, environmental degradation, and global food shortages, alongside some of the more implicit indications of racism, sexism, or homophobia that accompanied this flourishing conversation about family planning.

North Americans had historically maintained laws that restricted the use of contraception, despite deep pockets of support for coercive sterilization of some segments of the population, including people who were Indigenous, disabled, mentally ill, or poor.[4] In 1968, Stanford University professor Paul Ehrlich added to the conversation with an alarming exposé into the calamities of overpopulation. Ehrlich published *The Population Bomb*, in which he predicted that within a decade the world would face an unprecedented global famine resulting from overpopulation and insufficient food resources.[5] The predominant and most immediate areas of concern in Erlich's book were in China and India, where the population in each country had surpassed half a billion people.[6] Ehrlich forecasted disaster, and in doing so he helped to reinvigorate Malthusian ideas about mass starvation and population control that grabbed the attention of policy makers, religious authorities, environmentalists, and family planners around the globe, including in Canada.[7] At that time, Canada – with the world's second-largest land mass, at just under ten million square kilometres, and one of the largest food producers on the planet – represented just 0.58 per cent of the world's total population, with twenty million people. This historical moment nonetheless captured the imagination of the country's policy makers, religious authorities, and civil servants, who began to think about Canadian families in a global context, or at least to consider how global ideas about population burdens affected discussions and laws regarding Canadian family planning.

Ehrlich also made the issue personal, perhaps modelling how people might respond to this population burden. Ehrlich and his wife, Anne, decided after one child that he should have a vasectomy.[8] According to contemporary commentators, Ehrlich claimed that "voluntary sterilization is one of the best means of conservation open to us." David and Helen Wolfers, fellow family planning advocates in the 1970s, further described the issue as "the bizarre struggle for the vasa deferentia of conservationists, antipollution groups and population watchers on both sides of the Atlantic."[9] Pushing the matter beyond that of individuals or personal decisions, this conceptualization of birth control framed the issue as one of international urgency, with ramifications for reducing poverty and preserving the environment. For North Americans living with relatively abundant resources and in less densely populated environments than those in India or China, taking birth control or volunteering for sterilization allowed them to participate in global solutions, while acting locally.

Birth control awoke. It did so on a scale perhaps unimagined by the many women who carried placards demanding equality and who struggled to wrestle their biology into some kind of syncopation with patriarchy. The changing attitudes toward birth control and voluntary sterilization helped to alter the playing field for feminists agitating for gender equality, but it also contributed to reimagining the application of birth control on a larger scale. The threat of the population bomb effectively helped to convince men and conservatives – indeed, even the Catholic Church when it came to impoverished and densely populated regions – that the fear of overpopulation was real and that it could be minimized by persuading women and men that birth control was their contribution to the creation of a more stable future.[10] For some women, access to birth control was a much more personal matter, one that allowed women to make career *and* family choices, regardless of whether their use of the Pill saved the planet. Despite the different justifications for decriminalizing birth control, the combination of rising fears about population growth, western feminism, and responsible citizenship colluded in a moment that allowed for new political alliances.

Birth control in this moment offered a pragmatic solution to the looming global crisis of overpopulating the planet, and for some, limiting population growth was a more sustainable response than increasing the food supply. Western feminists may have agreed with these larger concerns, but for many of them it meant fighting their own patriarchal battles before they could then confidently and unhypocritically peddle their advice elsewhere.[11] Indeed, Ehrlich's own book begged for a more immediate feminist intervention. His wife, Anne, was originally listed as coauthor but the publishers felt that a pocket-sized book would sell better with a single author. Paul became that author. Fifty years later, he admitted that he too was "a good example of male chauvinism back in those days."[12] Despite the fact that his wife went on to become a well-known author and collaborator in her own right, which he readily celebrates, the timing and symbolism of this outcome is a fitting entry point into a historical contextualization of population control and its complicated, and at times contradictory, relationship with western feminism.

Challenging Choices is a historical examination of how competing discourses on global population control, poverty, feminism, personal autonomy, race, and gender shaped reproductive politics in 1970s Canada. We suggest the 1970s were a pivotal moment in the changing discourse on birth control and sterilization: from the decriminalization of contraception in 1969 when the government seemingly made good on its promise to pull the state out of the bedrooms of the nation, up to the introduction of the Charter of Rights and Freedoms in 1982, which closely coincided with the recognition of the AIDS epidemic and a moral panic over sexually transmitted diseases that accompanied a backlash against liberal attitudes toward unmarried sex. During this decade, conversations about the legal and moral use of birth control shifted from an issue of prohibition to one of permission and even encouragement. Part of the predominant rationale for using birth control, at least in the public discourse, also changed from preventing degeneration to addressing concerns of global security. By the end of the 1970s it shifted again, as legal access to birth control became a symbol of what modern feminist activism could accomplish and was ultimately tied to a larger movement of human rights and gender equality.

The decision to decriminalize contraception overturned a law that was nearly eighty years old and challenged much more long-standing moral and cultural values. That it happened in the era of the campaigns for civil rights, sexual liberation, and other progressive causes perhaps made it seem less like the dramatic reversal that it was. The timing and context have shaped the historical narrative of reproductive rights in Canada, leading to an understanding of the 1970s as a short bridge between the rights-based claims of the 1960s and the eventual enshrinement of individual Charter rights in 1982. In fact, the rationales behind the decriminalization of birth control and discussion of its use in the 1970s were not individual rights-based arguments but arguments rooted in the idea of a greater good. Close attention to the policy discourse in this period reveals that consideration and care for the individual reproductive rights of Canadians were regularly subordinated to discussions about the impact of birth control on health and social services, the moral teaching of churches, the fiscal capacity of governments, and Canada's international aid aspirations. Conversations about family planning became entangled with discussions about the national economy and global overpopulation, leading to confusion and contradiction about the rights and responsibilities of citizenship. These conversations happened in an environment of latent (sometimes overt) racist, sexist, homophobic, classist, and ableist attitudes, which, as we will explore in this book, led to the unequal treatment of people and unequal access to reproductive rights and services.

The 1970s were also an important decade for Canada as it took its place on the international stage. Canadians joined a global conversation about population control that revisited older ideas about eugenics, heredity, and degeneration. Birth control, as a matter of choice, had always been part of the conversations on eugenics, but by at least the 1960s that conversation began to change. New medical technologies introduced during this period, namely the birth control pill, alongside new expectations for healthcare access after the introduction of Medicare, altered the playing field for discussions about medical interventions in reproductive health, who should have access to them, and who should be subjected to them. The projections about global food shortages not only put the spotlight on birth control as a viable response but also directed attention to Canada as a major food-producing nation, poised to contribute to global solutions. For nearly a century female-centred birth control had been legally prohibited; its use was reserved for population groups who were designated as suffering due to poverty, mental illness, or both. This patronizing approach gradually changed over the course of the twentieth century, but we argue that many of same principles lingered into the 1970s as Canadian authorities discussed the merits of decriminalizing contraception. The early debates about eugenics in the 1910s and 1920s shared a common theme with the birth control discussions in the 1960s and 1970s: economics and abstract ideas about the collective good took priority over moral, cultural, or social commitments to the value of individual lives. Birth control was not yet a debate about choice as much as it was a debate about cost.

The financial cost of birth control came as a price tag for establishing healthcare services, especially in Canada's northern regions. Costs were also involved in prohibiting and policing birth control and, consequently, investing in child welfare services, foster care programs, and homes for unwed mothers. The expansion of services in the post–World War II era meant that provisions for family allowances, maternity leave benefits, and lost labour resulting from an increased number of women in the workplace taking leave to care for children all added up to create financial implications for a welfare-state bureaucracy.[13]

The cost of decriminalizing birth control, however, went well beyond dollar figures. If global population numbers continued to increase at projected rates, birth control technologies would proliferate in other regions while Canada, and many other western nations, continued to prohibit their use and failed to gain their share of the marketplace. Moreover, western leaders could not participate unhypocritically in promoting birth control abroad if they refused to discuss its use at home. Liberalizing the use of contraception at home, at least initially, served to help maintain traditional lines of authority more than disrupt them. The same logic extended into domestic spheres, whether it meant continuing to prioritize the superiority of heterosexual, married family decisions, or the primacy of the male decision-maker.[14] These power dynamics were poised to change again in the coming years, but we suggest that a close look at the 1970s helps to provide an understanding of continuity more than change.

Eugenics and birth control have shared an uneasy relationship historically and historiographically. Birth control was a central tenet of eugenic programs, but the historical literature has tended to separate the study of eugenics from the history of birth control.[15] Eugenics, defined by Francis Galton as "nobility in birth," emerged in the late nineteenth century amid a wave of enthusiasm for studies of evolution, heredity, and a science of biology that achieved new theoretical energy through Charles Darwin's work. Galton's intervention into this field put biology into direct conversation with family studies, invoking questions of heredity and animating debates over the relative influences of nature and nurture.[16] The notion of purposeful reproduction, whether through selective breeding typified by the work of Gregor Mendel or through prohibitions on reproduction as embraced by eugenics societies, made the study of eugenics a fertile area for exploring elements of reproduction, fertility, and governance.[17] Far beyond Galton's original, and perhaps slightly naïve, suggestion that good breeding, or elite couplings, could produce desirable qualities, eugenicists by the early twentieth century recognized that purposeful breeding, and selective breeding, could have distinct advantages for the efficient management of populations.

Canadian historians have tended to separate scholarship on eugenics before World War II from studies of birth control and abortion activism, especially as it gathers momentum in the second half of the twentieth century. Angus and Arlene McLaren pioneered these fields in Canada, first producing a comprehensive study of contraception and abortion in Canada between 1880 and 1980, a period characterized largely by prohibitions against controlling fertility that were held in place by law and religious authority.[18] Angus McLaren followed this up nearly a decade later with a groundbreaking study of eugenics in Canada from the 1910s to World War II. Historians of eugenics have reinforced this framing of eugenics as having ended with World War II, noting that Nazi Germany fundamentally altered the scale and scope of eugenics programs. Contemporary scientists and policy makers drew critical attention to the flawed pseudoscience of heredity and the faulty logic of eugenicists whose enthusiasm for targeting undesirable populations quickly overwhelmed any scientific rigour that may have theoretically underpinned their original intentions.[19] Despite the significant impact of World War II on changing attitudes toward eugenics, the theories and in some cases the programs themselves remained in place, becoming tangled up within the history of contraception and birth control.

The history of birth control, contraception, and abortion in Canada has attracted attention from legal scholars and social historians, chiefly those interested in how the laws activated social movements or discriminated against women through medico-legal means. More recently, scholars have looked beyond the specific legal dimensions and explored how women accessed abortion despite prohibitions and difficult access points or, conversely, how women continued to be victims of a paternalistic state.[20] The topic of abortion has also generated particular attention in the historical literature, again focusing in part on the legal parameters, and a close look at physician Henry Morgentaler, whose legal battles fundamentally altered the landscape for abortions in Canada. His public struggles to provide abortion in the 1980s drew concerted attention to the legal and social implications of abortion studies in Canada and inspired a body of literature in its wake.[21]

More recently, scholars studying trends outside of Canada especially have taken a step back from these debates, looking instead at larger trends or global concerns about population control, economics, and environmental concerns. Scholars including Ian Dowbiggin, Matthew Connelly, and Alison Bashford have argued convincingly that nation-states were ill equipped to handle the significance of birth control without looking beyond borders to appreciate the global economy of fertility.[22] In a focused study on how population control became a question suited for economists, historian Michelle Murphy investigated how the science of life became an economic object of fascination within the historical spectre of the population bomb. She explains that "lives not worth being born abstractly held a negative economic value that would be attached to the possible life of future people, particularly non-white people and poor people." She emphasizes that economizing life had significant implications for a global economic outlook that rationalized human life through such mathematical accounting. Moreover, the reliance on scientific indicators of the problems and solutions provided a veneer of objectivity and certainty that was used to legitimize population-control measures designed to target poor and brown populations by collapsing the categories of fertility and poverty into a single problem, while also elevating the technological conditions of fertility control with access to the world's resources. Murphy continues, "Out of these quantitative models a new way of distributing life chances and the value of life had been built that did not need to rely on biological race but could continue to re-enact racism. Some must not be born so that future others might prosper."[23] While economists tended to focus on the Global South, Canadian intellectuals and government planners nonetheless paid attention to the economics of birth control coupled with antipoverty strategies as they looked at their own national context and sought strategies for reducing poverty with minimal investments.

In *Challenging Choices*, we aim to frame Canadian decisions within these larger discussions by looking closely at how Canadian policy makers reconciled the changing tenor of birth control debates with a desire to maintain more traditional lines of authority at home. To do so, we attempt to lay bare some of the earlier debates about eugenics to understand how birth control fit into conversations aimed explicitly at population control in Canada, whether for people considered mentally unfit or for Indigenous women considered undesirable mothers. By concentrating on how the changes to contraception laws affected different subgroups of Canadians, we highlight some of the contradictions that continued to operate in the domain of birth control, which became a matter of choice for some and an act of coercion over others.

The cause of birth control appealed to early twentieth-century social reformers as a progressive response to a host of challenges associated with immigration, urbanization, and poverty. In North America, early feminists brandished birth control campaigns alongside those for suffrage. Birth control in this sense was usually not intended for the women agitating for the vote but instead part of a progressive response on behalf of women living in poverty.[24] In other words, more often than not, middle- and upper-class feminists (like the British expats Barbara and George Cadbury in Canada) supported birth control in a philanthropic gesture toward people living in poverty or those assumed to be feebleminded, expecting neither group to be capable of responsible parenthood. Mental hygiene movements swelled in North America in the late nineteenth and early twentieth centuries, promising to address the growing ranks of mentally unfit people from overwhelming the population through careless and rampant reproduction and a disproportionate drain on the nation-building agenda.[25] Stemming this tide became part of a progressive response to human suffering, and birth control when applied to these populations appeared magnanimous and just.

Between 1945 and 1969, Canadian scholarship suggests that agitation for birth control, as a matter of choice, became more subtle or even moved underground. McLaren and McLaren suggest that despite clear evidence that many Canadian families were practising some form of contraception in the first half of the twentieth century, public discussions on the topic tended to regard it as "problematic"; they argue that it "was associated in the public mind either with sexual radicals on the far left or with reactionary Malthusians on the far right." They go on to say that birth control discourse was "rescued" by feminists who later brought respectability to the topic, but the public discourse on birth control remained rather coded.[26]

Prior to 1960, women in North America had limited options for birth control technology. The first oral contraceptive, Enovid, was approved by the US Food and Drug Administration in 1960 and became available in Canada the following year. American historian Liz Watkins describes how at that time diaphragms and spermicides could be obtained through a pharmacist, and condoms were available over the counter. Otherwise, couples resorted to withdrawal, douching, and rhythm methods, all of which are unreliable.[27] Regardless of the existence of birth control technologies, their legality also remained in question. In Canada, the law stipulated that "everyone is guilty of an indictable offence and liable to two years' imprisonment who knowingly, without lawful excuse or justification, offers to sell, advertises, publishes an advertisement of or has for sale or disposal of any medicine, drug or article intended or represented as a means of preventing conception or causing abortion."[28] The Criminal Code of Canada set out this prohibition in 1892, long before Enovid existed. The Canadian laws relaxed in 1969, but already in the 1960s advertisements about the birth control pill began appearing in medical journals, suggesting that the law had fallen out of sync with attitudes and practices. Heather Molyneaux discovered that the *Canadian Medical Association Journal* (*CMAJ*) began advertising the birth control pill as early as 1961 and she recognized that in some cases birth control information had been circulating in relatively known channels, including through the Parent's Information Bureau in Ontario, suggesting that the 1892 prohibition on advertising birth control methods was no longer being policed.[29]

It was not until the 1960s that the issue of birth control significantly resurfaced in the public, appearing in newspapers and in medical texts as a viable option for limiting family size and thereby chipping away at the earlier pronatalist arguments about how best to plan Canadian families. The introduction of the birth control pill in 1960 attracted attention as a feat of science and even a challenge to nature.[30] This phase in the history of birth control incorporated new technologies, reached new populations, and acquired new advocates. Historians too have been alert to the different conceptualizations of birth control, either focusing on its relationship to eugenics before World War II or emphasizing its reemergence in the 1960s with a different set of connotations. Canadian scholars have not fully reconciled how the issue of population control in the 1960s interrupted domestic discussions about birth control, never mind the more subtle practices of child separation, coercive sterilization, or institutional segregation that all play into histories of family formation.

Indeed, when the Canadian Parliament amended the Criminal Code in 1969 to finally legalize birth control, New Democratic Party (NDP) member Grace MacInnis, an ardent supporter of women's rights and access to birth control, lauded Bill C-150 particularly for the opportunity it gave Canada to join the (western) world community to control Third World populations. Canada, she argued, was hypocritical in advocating birth control abroad while keeping it illegal at home; "the people of other countries ... could always say to us 'Aha! You want us as dark-skinned people to control our population but you yourself cannot practice birth control legally.' We can now help the peoples of these countries freely and openly."[31] In September 1970, the federal government authorized the Canadian International Development Agency to make major contributions to the United Nations Fund for Population Activities and the International Planned Parenthood Federation (IPPF).[32]

Within the span of only a few years, the personal act of restricting fertility exploded onto the international stage as a major political issue poised to address a whole host of global economic and environmental crises. The United Nations convened its first World Population Conference in Bucharest, Romania, in 1974, where 136 nations, including Canada, represented by 1,400 delegates, renewed Malthusian concerns on a global scale. As western nations peeled back their restrictions on access to birth control, many western feminists celebrated what they saw as a triumph of their collective civil protests against many patriarchal societies that held women captive to their biology. But, the spectre of population control required a series of uncomfortable alliances and exposed some of the inherent contradictions regarding who indeed was considered responsible for planning Canadian families. Population control became a rallying cry for progressive reformers from the left, but it also made good fiscal sense, which appealed to broadly held conservative perspectives that had more often been resistant to birth control.

By the 1970s, eugenic philosophies from the nineteenth and early twentieth centuries had mutated and found new currency and became firmly embedded in discussions about reproductive choice and humanitarian aid. The bodies targeted directly as the sites of birth control became targets for discussions about the relationship between poverty and fertility control, regardless of any concern for population density. Foucauldian concepts of discipline and governmentality course through this subject area, once again illustrating how capillaries of power colluded to make populations bend to new ideological frameworks of what was considered progressive, and modern, but often subversive.[33] The seemingly new political motivations that divided the politics of reproduction along the axis of rich and poor, developed and underdeveloped, or North and South, continued to represent fundamental and abiding conflicts over issues of autonomy, sovereignty, resources, and health. Mainstream western feminists celebrated the decriminalization of contraception and abortion as a progressive step toward individual autonomy and a significant improvement in women's capacity to engage in family planning. Governments, however, struggled to balance the macro concerns of population control with growing demands for reproductive health services within an increasingly expensive welfare state. The clash of global, national, and individual concerns about family planning produced significant tensions over how to respond to competing demands from local communities seeking individual autonomy and public health services.

Challenging Choices suggests that eugenics and birth control were never fully delinked during this period, creating complicated alliances, confusing characterizations of what was indeed progressive, and leading to differential treatment in the provision or restriction of birth control. We acknowledge that birth control has been used across the ideological spectrum to spur competing visions for progress. We argue that traditional Canadian authorities – that is, lawmakers, religious leaders, and civil servants – recognized an opportunity to embrace birth control as a pragmatic solution to global problems and moreover as a strategic way to bring Canada into that solution; we suggest too that despite these changes, embracing birth control in the 1970s also allowed authorities to maintain some aspects of the status quo. That is to say, despite the dominant characterization of the 1960s as a period of upheaval, revolution, and shifting Canadian identities, we argue that the 1970s represents a period of continuity when it came to maintaining the paternalistic nature of the Canadian state.[34] Traditional authorities remained in positions of power, be that the male-dominated halls of Canadian Parliament or the colonial framework of settler-Indigenous relations or the heteronormative values associated with family planning and sexuality.

Reproductive politics in the 1970s readily invoke an interpretation that emphasizes a narrative of liberation. The Age of Aquarius, popularly associated with the 1960s and 1970s, captured a sense of New Age ideas, a culmination of hippie and counterculture critiques of power and authority, and a celebration of the triumph of civil rights that created new horizons for equality in the workplace as well as in the bedroom.[35] The 1970s was a decade poised to enjoy the rewards of postwar struggles to bring women into the workplace, to confront differences in race and gender in the classroom, and to reap the benefits of the welfare state. Unfortunately for many people, the promised bounty was not altogether forthcoming; human rights, pay equity, and sexual liberation did not immediately overturn more entrenched cultural practices of racism, homophobia, or sexism. Successive recessions in that decade also strained state infrastructure and clawed back some of the services that had blossomed in a postwar era of reconstruction and growth.

Popular media representations have illustrated this period with images of confident young women, characteristically unshackled from their bras but also liberated by new technologies, labour-saving devices, and now the legal right to exercise those new freedoms through the science of family planning. With new technologies and old, women could take their places in higher education and the professions without pregnancy and child rearing threatening to undermine their performance in the workplace.[36] Or so it seemed. This interpretation captures only one aspect of the relationship between the state and family planning. Far from simply creating a new marketplace for reproductive services, the changes beginning in the 1970s altered the culture of reproductive politics by repoliticizing family planning within a framework of middle-class, "healthy," and heteronormative values.

Relaxing laws on birth control helped to animate the second-wave feminist movement as women demanded access to paid employment and higher education, claiming that they could control their bodies and plan when to have children. Feminists raised the ire of traditional authorities, some of whom engaged in debates over birth control as a mechanism for protecting the sanctity of the family or, put differently, to retain the patriarchal status quo. Some of the more obvious religious and political divisions continued to frame the terms of the debates.[37] Yet new alliances and detractors also emerged in the changing landscape amid contests over family values, same-sex marriages, sex-selection technologies, and cross-border adoptions, all of which contributed to a (re)defining of the modern family.

These contests also gave rise to the vocabulary of "choice": the idea that women, and later men, could choose to have children and could plan those births to coordinate with their own education and career options. Debates about choice have collapsed into more simplistic categories of "pro-life" and "pro-choice," which serves to further gloss over other cultural factors that shape the modern family, while ignoring some of the earlier history that gave rise to notions of choice within a more conservative framework. In this book, therefore, we self-consciously move away from these dichotomous categories, and the historical divisions between illegal contraception and legal contraception marked by the formal laws, and instead highlight examples that cut across these rather more basic categories. We argue that the legal changes affected Canadians differently depending on other social, cultural, religious, and health conditions. In complicating the story by focusing on bodies that are routinely excluded from the progressive, reformist discourse, we show that for some groups of people the legal changes did not in fact bring about an era of reproductive liberty but instead reinforced traditional power dynamics and authoritative structures.

We identify four categories that warrant sustained analysis: Indigenous women, women and men with intellectual and physical disabilities, men, and teenage girls. By bringing these perspectives into the conversation, we hope that a different picture emerges. Many of these voices articulated an alternative set of challenges for individuals who faced new levels of government regulation or state intervention as they negotiated their reproductive health, rights, and responsibilities in the so-called era of sexual liberation. Importantly, their experiences help to illustrate that there are many ways to plan a modern family and many ways in which the concept of life was pitted against choice to create a new moral landscape for evaluating classic questions of population control. Our book sheds new light on this complicated relationship among eugenics, birth control, and population control in Canada, locating these changes within a global movement that involved discussions about balancing resources, human rights, and national development.

CASE STUDIES

Indigenous Women

During the 1970s, reproductive bodies that fell outside of the typical family planning model – middle class, heteronormative, urban – experienced a different set of choices when it came to birth control. Indigenous women faced particular challenges compared with the options available to urban, non-Indigenous women seeking contraception and abortions; these challenges and the policy response to them are the subject of chapters 2 and 3. The poverty of choices, particularly in underserviced regions in northern Canada, reveals how access to reproductive rights was profoundly shaped by class, race, and region. In many Indigenous communities, health services were minimal or nonexistent, requiring women to travel great distances for standard care or do without. Alongside these physical barriers were the catastrophic legacies of the assimilative policies of the Canadian government toward Indigenous peoples, which had been calculated to break down families and sever ties between generations. Indigenous family planning did not readily fit the profile of a 1970s middle-class settler family, particularly when considered against the backdrop of claims of genocide levied at the government during this period. Fertility and sovereignty overlapped in complicated ways, with a Red Power movement burgeoning as Indigenous Canadians crafted their own political movements in Canada, stimulating a different kind of reproductive activism aimed instead at having, and keeping, children.[38] Population growth and Indigenous family planning efforts redirected attention away from contraception and abortion and instead demanded services that desegregated health services and supported Indigenous women's choices to build healthy families on their own terms.

Yet Indigenous people did not all share the same vision for family planning. Indigenous women debated one another and fought to be heard, by other feminists as well as within their own communities. Women in northern Canada, for example, demanded better services in their communities and resented having to travel hundreds of kilometres south to access basic maternal and infant care. The federal government, reluctant to build health services in the North, rationalized that it was cheaper to move patients to hospitals. Restricting local services also ensured that women left their homes and community networks to receive reproductive health care where they could be closely monitored.

Indigenous women living in Canadian provinces confronted different kinds of challenges. Residential schools continued to operate in some areas, while the legacy of trauma, abuse, and forced removal of children from their families reverberated through the generations.[39] The Sixties' Scoop – the forced removal of Indigenous children from their families and their adoption by non-Indigenous families – likewise left deep emotional scars on communities and continued in certain forms through the 1970s.[40] The rising enthusiasm for birth control and family planning had first to confront this legacy of injustice and the belief that Indigenous families were somehow ill suited to raise their own children. Having and keeping children at home became a priority as these communities struggled to rebuild after losing generations of their children. Recent findings from the Truth and Reconciliation Commission of Canada underscore the horrific conditions that children faced in the Indian residential school system, resulting in widespread illness, poor nutrition, and death. Confronting colonialism in these communities had specific repercussions for family planning, which did not coincide with reducing family size. Rather, in this context, many Indigenous women sought to exercise a different set of choices: those related to raising their own healthy children.

In spite of the federal government's claims to be pulling the state out of the bedrooms of Canadians with its 1969 legal amendments, for Indigenous women the state became more invested in their reproductive bodies than ever before. For these women, embracing reproductive choice was not an exercise in personal freedom but a politically loaded decision, and it raised questions specific to their contexts: for instance, the *choice* to have and keep children in the family rather than surrender them into a residential school system or a system of child welfare and adoption services. The *choice* to leave their communities and support networks in order to access hospital services, including pre- and postnatal care that sometimes entailed months away from husbands, other children, and extended families. Or, Indigenous women could exercise the *choice* to align themselves with the more vocal male activists in the rising tide of Red Power activism. Indigenous rights movements in the 1970s embraced the discourse of sovereignty, with its embedded connotations of pronatalism, as part of a larger reaction to colonial power imbalances. Choosing Indigenous sovereignty also had more specific implications for Indigenous feminists whose articulation of motherwork, with its explicit challenge to western conceptualizations of gender and its links to power, made the decision to restrict fertility a very different political act than the kinds of choices that non-Indigenous abortion activists demanded. The threatening spectre of a global population bomb extended to Canadian regions as poverty and race collided, realigning the priorities of population control with colonialization.

By looking closely at federal government and Indian Health Services (IHS) records, we examine how policy makers addressed these questions and demands for improved healthcare services in Indigenous communities. We review correspondence to reveal which voices or influences captured the most attention and how civil servants responded in a manner that both emphasized minimizing expenditures and appropriated the language of choice or responsibility to support their own agenda of cost containment. We are critical of the way that policy makers and bureaucrats seized upon the hypothetical international crisis of global overpopulation to design a set of healthcare options that suited their political and economic needs. We look at how this process unfolded and show how it meant ignoring the realities faced by people "on the ground." To build our case, we focus primarily on the subjects of our critique and the sources they created, including government departmental records, public statements by politicians and civil servants, and internal memoranda and communications. The incorporation of testimony from people's lived experience would bolster our argument but also dilute the critique. Instead, we show that despite the evident need for improved health services, which was demonstrated in published reports, newspaper coverage, and public demonstrations, policy makers privileged a different set of priorities when designing the system.

Women and Men with Intellectual and Physical Disabilities

Another category of fertile bodies that posed challenges to liberal discourse on choice were already familiar to state authorities. Institutionalized individuals, classified as mentally, intellectually, or physically disabled, attracted specific attention in the context of population-control debates during the 1970s and are the subject of chapter 4. Many of these individuals had long been under severe restrictions, required as they were to live in long-stay custodial facilities. People with mental and intellectual disorders were among

Canadians most likely to have been sterilized through eugenics programs. In the 1970s, as those programs formally ended, psychiatric facilities also underwent a paradigmatic change in care, from a system that prioritized institutionalization to one that emphasized the benefits of care in the community. However, moving thousands of people into communities also raised concerns about promiscuity and sexual abuse, particularly for individuals already targeted as dependent or as incapable of independent living. Regardless of the reality of their capabilities, legislators, social workers, psychiatrists, and politicians debated the merits of allowing reproductive choice for individuals who continued to be viewed as incapable parents and, in some cases, dependent and often infantilized adults.[41] The twinned concerns of genetic disorders and assumptions about personal limitations fuelled debates that reached the Supreme Court of Canada about who has the right to decide the reproductive future of a person with a disability.[42]

Sifting through the legal debates, as well as the discussions raised by medical associations and government representatives in Ontario, we look at how decision-makers continued in the 1970s to exert authority over disabled bodies. Looking closely at correspondence among staff from custodial facilities for adults with mental and physical disabilities, we consider how staff, politicians, and parents of disabled children and adults attempted to retain their decision-making power over people considered incapable of responsible parenting.

Men

We think it is finally time to bring men into the history of reproductive rights activism; they are the subject of chapter 5. Middle-class married men in North America did not pursue vasectomies as a form of birth control en masse until the late 1960s and early 1970s. Vasectomy surgery was well understood among medical professionals by the turn of the twentieth century, but it remained primarily confined to use in institutional populations as part of population-control exercises, which was more in keeping with traditional sterilization and eugenic practices. For married women, sexual sterilization arose as a procedure that brought emancipation and autonomy from the burden of unwanted reproduction. For middle-class men, the vasectomy initially suggested a challenge to masculinity or an affront to manhood; over the course of the 1950s and 1960s, however, this attitude slowly changed. As birth control became a more openly discussed topic, and especially as women's contraceptive methods came under public scrutiny, the vasectomy operation emerged as a safer, cheaper, and arguably more efficient option for middle-class family planning than invasive surgeries or daily consumption of birth control pills for women.[43]

Men as fathers have not typically been part of the literature on birth control, yet their roles and the history of vasectomies is an important part of this discussion. Men appear more often than women as decision-makers, whether as bureaucrats or politicians or as presumed familial breadwinners, reinforcing the notion that family planning and rearing is still shaped by men's decisions. Individual men, like businessman and eugenics supporter A.R. Kaufman, who appears in chapter 5, play a historically significant role in promoting birth control, though Kaufman emerges in this history amid a set of contradictions, acting in ways that appear both progressive and patronizing. Paying close attention to how masculinity is performed in this context helps to illustrate how men have participated in birth control activism and, later, how men embraced vasectomies in their own attempts to develop masculine responses to population control and family planning.

Beginning in the late 1960s, individual men put pressure on medical authorities to provide vasectomies. An inquiry into five Ontario hospitals in 1967 revealed that elective sterilization surgeries on males had been taking place and produced tricky legal challenges. Ontario's physicians argued that if patients provided informed consent, the surgery should be considered legal. Since male patients sought the operation for contraceptive purposes, however, it raised other issues within the Criminal Code about the use of birth control. Although the 1892 Criminal Code prohibited the use of any contraceptive devices, alongside abortion, it made no explicit mention of male contraception per se. Nonetheless, surgeons worried that they could be charged with assault under this law, regardless of consent.[44]

In 1970, Donald J. Dodds, former president of Planned Parenthood of Toronto and a general practitioner who had served in Toronto, Montreal, Boston, Halifax, and Curling, Newfoundland, published a small booklet describing his experiences with male sterilization. After performing his own vasectomy he had offered the procedure to other men. He attributed the rise in popularity of the vasectomy to the publicity surrounding the birth control pill. At first, the Pill brought discussions of birth control out in the open, and by the late 1960s those discussions included consideration of the Pill's severe and damaging potential side effects, ranging from migraines and blood clots to aneurisms and even death. Vasectomies, in contrast, had fewer reported risks or side effects.[45]

Young Women

Young women were also the subject of debates – specifically, as to whether reproductive choice should trickle down to young, unmarried girls and women under the age of twenty – and are the focus of chapter 6. Teenage girls seeking abortions furnished anti-abortion activists with gruesome images of broken morals and a country in ruin. Meanwhile, pro-choice activists remained uncomfortable with abortion when it seemed to replace contraception. When it came to unmarried teens, contraception, or, better yet, abstinence, was still preferred. This logic further underscored a long-held conviction that reproductive choices were reserved for responsible individuals, and part of being responsible meant delaying sexual encounters until heterosexual marriage.

Throughout the 1970s, as abortion attracted considerable media and public attention in the wake of its decriminalization, the abortion debate also focused the morals of parenthood – or rather, single motherhood – on young women. Pregnant, unmarried teenage girls emerged as the most alarming category of individuals seeking abortions. Their youth and (predominantly) unmarried status signalled sexual promiscuity and fuelled the claims of anti-abortionists that such operations merely contributed to moral and social decay. While many Canadians celebrated the retreat of the state from the bedrooms of married couples in good health, the state began developing strategies for implementing more extensive networks of surveillance over young and unmarried female bodies.

Monitoring abortions was facilitated by the requirement that all women seeking abortions had to first go before a therapeutic abortion committee (TAC), a procedure that was codified with the change in the law and that quickly became one of the most controversial provisions of the abortion law. The records of the TACs in Calgary and Edmonton, combined with letters from obstetricians, reveal how the public debates about abortion and a woman's right to choose overshadowed the more pernicious practice of sterilizing women and aborting fetuses from women deemed unfit for parenting. Obstetricians and hospital administrators were caught in a contradiction: on the one hand, upset by the rising tide of "abortion on demand," which they connected with irresponsible middle-class feminists who challenged traditional family values and over which the physicians attempted to regain medical authority; and on the other hand, less conflicted about proceeding with abortions, in combination with or separate from tubal ligations, on women and teenage girls whom they considered incapable of the responsibilities of parenthood. In other words, some in the medical community seemed inclined to provide abortions for unmarried teens more out of concern for their future well-being as mothers and taxpaying citizens than out of fear that they were otherwise destined to be economically draining recipients of social service benefits. Those same medical authorities, however, did not extend this consideration to married women, who they felt abused the abortion law to satisfy selfish desires to limit family size, implying that they were shirking their duty of raising responsible children. The issue of choice in this context had effectively absorbed an essential grain of earlier eugenic philosophy and continued to rely on the authority of the medical profession to determine who made good parents, either biologically or socially.

In order to track these debates about teenage pregnancies, sex education, and abortion counselling services, we looked to how this topic was described in Canadian newspapers. We first sampled regional discussions and then focused on hotspots in Canada, especially the Atlantic and Prairie Provinces; both regions claimed to have the highest rates of teen pregnancy. Tracing this issue through medical journals, we then compared newspaper coverage with medical responses, finding that both converged around concerns for long-term poverty and dependence as the ultimate reason for permitting teen abortions.

Challenging Choices adds a new dimension to the historical conversation on reproductive health by bringing together perspectives that are traditionally left out of histories of reproductive politics in Canada. By demonstrating a longer history of contested reproductive politics, we defy a simplistic "life" or "choice" conceptualization and instead emphasize the multiple social, cultural, economic, and political factors that have shaped family planning discourse into the twenty-first century. The 1970s represent an important moment for bringing some of these discussions into the public domain, but ultimately, we argue that many of the dominant power dynamics remained in place, continuing to limit the choices available to many Canadians. By contextualizing these choices, we hope also to contribute to a deeper, perhaps more complex and inclusive understanding of a diversity of family values.

CHAPTER ONE

Making a New Mainstream

In 1967, Minister of Justice Pierre Elliott Trudeau, who would soon become the prime minister of Canada, famously remarked that "the state has no business in the bedrooms of the nation."[1] He made this statement as part of a move to introduce landmark legislation that would decriminalize contraception, abortion, and homosexuality. The gesture symbolically represented a reversal of a set of legal, moral, and medical codes that had been in place for nearly a century. The changes reinforced the idea that a significant liberalizing agenda was at work, spearheaded by activists and soon to be captured in the Liberals' 1968 election campaign slogan, "A Just Society." In making such a declaration, Trudeau positioned himself as an astute observer of cultural trends and a champion of diversity in a modern, civilized world.

Yet, even when the bill was first proposed, other parliamentarians questioned the superficiality of the claim that decriminalization of specific sexual acts would necessarily bring about a separation of bedroom and state. Progressive Conservative member Robert McCleave suggested, "We have here an attempt to separate the law from personal morality or, as has been stated by the architect of the so-called just society, the state has no place in the nation's bedrooms. That statement has a rather motto-like note ring to it. But I suggest ... that the state does have a place in the nation's bedrooms." Indeed, with the expansion of government services, from family allowances to income tax, immigration laws to disability supports, McCleave was perhaps correct to cleverly suggest that in fact the proverbial Canadian bedroom was already "pretty crowded."[2]

The parliamentary debates over contraception and abortion are important as much for how they illustrate the tenor of the conversation over how to craft the legal reforms as for what they reveal about significant gaps and blind spots in these discussions. Parliamentarians, who were designing the laws, were demonstrably out of touch with the conversations taking place outside of Parliament at the time they proposed the new laws. Contrasting those debates with the citizens' letters and public discussions prompted by the contemporaneous Royal Commission on the Status of Women reveals deep contradictions in how the issue of family planning was presented to Canadians. The discourse around reproductive rights in these two formal public arenas diverged dramatically depending on the location of the conversation and the position of the speaker.

Despite the suggestion that Canadians now had more government services implicated in their family planning decisions, the legal changes regarding the Criminal Code were significant. Since 1892, based on British common law, birth control, contraception, abortion, and same-sex activities had been criminalized and punishable by jail time. Reducing the moral judgment on and legal punishment for these activities and instead acknowledging such behaviours as a feature of modern society, not to mention an issue of personal autonomy, was not, however, without its complications. Despite Trudeau's famous quip, the state in fact remained concerned with what was going on in many Canadian bedrooms. This chapter explores some of the intellectual, medical, and cultural dynamics that animated these debates at the end of the 1960s as Canadian society debated reform to particular features of the Criminal Code that promised to reconcile past injustices by overturning discriminatory prohibitions. A closer look at the realities of reproductive rights since the 1970s reveals a much more complicated picture of modern reproductive health and family planning than one that simply celebrates a new era of modern reproduction, freed from state surveillance.

We begin this chapter by looking at how Canadians talked publicly about family planning, if at all. By the time this issue was being actively debated in Parliament, beginning in 1967, Canadians had already been exposed to competing rationales for using birth control: during a eugenics era to control feeblemindedness, as a response to poverty during the economic depression, and increasingly by the 1960s as a safe medical intervention that aided in a more strategic form of family planning.

EUGENICS IN CANADA

In the 1920s and 1930s most Canadian jurisdictions entertained eugenics laws.[3] Alberta introduced Canada's first Sexual Sterilization Act in 1928, and British Columbia followed in 1933. While many provinces debated, and nearly implemented, similar laws, these western provinces were the only two that formally practised eugenics, through programs that both provinces maintained until the 1970s. These early programs, which concentrated their efforts on sexual sterilization surgeries for people considered mentally or physically disabled, remained closely tied to a history of institutionalization.[4] Eugenic sterilizations continued in the post–World War II period and assumed that certain individuals were a genetic risk to the population. Moreover, candidates for these surgeries were deemed incapable of responsible parenthood for either hereditary or sociocultural reasons.

In Alberta, sterilizations were performed without obtaining consent from individuals who were considered "mentally deficient." Contraception laws, therefore, did not apply equally to people considered genetically or intellectually incapable of "responsible parenthood." Conversely, contraception, including sexual sterilization operations and abortions, among middle-class and allegedly healthy families remained illegal until 1969. By the end of World War II, however, families that had expanded to or beyond their financial and emotional capacity were increasingly resorting to creative methods of obtaining physician-assisted, permanent contraception by challenging the eugenic laws in western Canada.[5] Some jurisdictions even accounted for women who had reached a point of emotional exhaustion, sometimes described merely as weakness, or psychological distress, caused by multiple births.

Although the 1970s are recognized as the time when reproductive choice shifted to actions connoting individual autonomy, the decade also involved rebranding the instruments of contraception and introducing new technologies of individual control, namely the birth control pill. The medical technologies required to perform surgical sterilizations, provide temporary contraception, or produce abortions had a longer history, but one that was implicated with coercive surgeries that implied the outright denial of individual autonomy and a dark past of attempts at nonconsensual population control. Indeed, during the 1970s the discourse on birth control often retained the language, laws, and technologies of eugenics but at the same time embraced an emerging discourse of reproductive autonomy. "Choice" became a key concept, shorthand for progress, humanitarianism, and, of course, feminism. But the context of that choice was complicated by long-standing tensions involving race, gender, class, and place. The notion of reproductive choice, with its focus on access to abortion, is less useful when one considers the eugenic policies aimed at Indigenous, minority, and disabled women. More appropriate is the term "reproductive justice," or access to the range of choices that includes abortion but also the choice to become pregnant, to have access to one's own midwife, and to raise children in healthy circumstances.[6]

By the end of the 1960s the moral compass had rotated, from a direction when preventing fertility was considered backward and counterproductive to one when the reverse was true. Yet, for those whose choices went against the tide, their bodies continued to be marred as counterproductive, backward, and in need of paternalistic intervention to protect or control their decisions for their own good. Rejecting birth control, which had initially been a badge of moral honour, became a symbol of backward thinking. Put differently, government planners believed that resisting birth control created a new public health problem: that of endemic poverty, poor health outcomes, and economic dependence, all features that necessitated government intervention.

In the 1970s, several nations were coming to grips with the controversial relationship between eugenics and birth control. Nation-states and individuals remained locked in a contest over who has the right to control fertility. The discussion changed shape as laws throughout the western world increasingly decriminalized contraception and abortion, even while the vocal authorities of the Roman Catholic Church remained steadfast in their resistance to these manoeuvres. As we have seen in the work of Gisela Bock, Laura Briggs, and others, however, Catholic women did not always heed these prohibitions and by the 1970s were adopting birth control in numbers similar to their non-Catholic counterparts.[7] Feminists brandished the new laws as landmark achievements in a human rights discourse that celebrated individual rights over state priorities or religious morality; one might even argue that these feminists cherished this moment as a triumph over institutions of misogyny and patriarchy. As historians Georgina Feldberg and Judy Walzer Leavitt have also shown, these political shifts created changes in doctor-patient encounters, with more women entering medicine and more research dollars invested in obstetrics and gynecology. By the mid-twentieth century the vast majority of births took place in hospitals, under the watchful eyes of physicians and nurses and with ready access to emergency services and postnatal care.[8]

The history of contraception laws does not fully reveal how family planning occurred during an era of contraceptive prohibition, nor does that legal history capture how the cultural and moral discourse shifted throughout the twentieth century. When Canadians turned to their legal institutions to change the laws, the gesture may have seemed salutary or even outdated.

The parliamentary debates surrounding the 1969 amendment occupied politicians for nearly eighteen months of political discussion. Over those many months, the tenor of the debates covered a lot of ground, but much of it did not in fact focus on questions of women's autonomy or the language of reproductive rights later taken up by women reacting to the changes in the law. Indeed, by comparing the contemporaneous conversations inside Parliament, in the heavily male-dominated government offices, with the discussions and submissions taking place across Canada as part of the Royal Commission on the Status of Women, dominated by women's voices, we reveal a very different set of conversations. The fact that both conversations converged on the issue of contraception and its decriminalization as a key point for moving forward helps to illustrate how decision-makers incorporated elements of progressive discourse into their decision to change the legislation. By looking closely at the parliamentary debates, however, we also suggest that the decisions were based not on concerns for the welfare of women, nor on recognition of patriarchal structures; instead, the legislative decisions altered the laws to achieve goals that supported a more conservative agenda.

Canadians may have been somewhat surprised by the contents of the 1967 proposed legislation. Birth control was already being provided through some public health agencies across the country, suggesting that its legal prohibition was already out of sync with popular practice; the legal amendment, then, might simply bring law in line with practice.[9] Indeed, provincial health services were in some regions complicit in distributing birth control information, contrary to the provisions of the law. Moreover, news coverage of the issue seemed to demand that the government take more, not less, control over the issue, whether that control resulted from assuming leadership on global population control or taking a firm stance on providing health services that reduced a reliance on illegal abortions. The philosophical motivations for decriminalization, however, were much more diverse than the outcome has suggested.

Big city papers like the *Toronto Star* reported in April 1967, before the bill was introduced, that efforts by the government to establish family planning clinics in Ontario "should certainly win public approval." The article went on to suggest that birth control had become rather mainstream and that the challenge now was really about removing the last vestiges of prohibition so that everyone had unencumbered access: "Too often in the past the well-to-do have had access to birth control information and devices while the poor and less educated mothers have not known where to turn ... Any woman, whether an immigrant mother with little English or a troubled adolescent from a gilded home, should be able to find out where to go for advice and help." Indeed, the article continued, "even the Roman Catholic Church now concedes that governments have a social responsibility to promote population control."[10] This claim would become more controversial the following year, when the Pope reconfirmed the Catholic position in *Humanae Vitae*, yet at least according to the *Toronto Star* birth control had become part of modern living. Removing the legal barriers to contraception and abortion was therefore framed by some as a humanitarian deed, bringing these technologies to underserviced populations.

This purportedly humanitarian interpretation had a much deeper history of coercive population control, forced sterilization, and eugenic programs that targeted vulnerable people on account of their race, presumed intelligence, physical health, and socioeconomic status.[11] Throughout the first part of the twentieth century, eugenics in North America targeted individuals primarily in poor communities, many of whom were also racialized or suffered from other health risks.[12] Eugenics advocates had long wrestled with the moral dilemma of identifying who was fit to reproduce and had traditionally been more cautious about promoting birth control for middle and upper classes owing to long-standing fears of degeneration. Birth control itself was not the problem; rather, it was the apparent fecundity among poor people and the general inability to plan families scientifically, and with confidence, that sat at the heart of debates over human fertility.

By the late 1960s, those concerns remained at play in the context of birth control but had also gathered political momentum, as family planning became linked to women's equal rights. Equal rights in this context referred to access to full, independent, and secure economic employment. Removing the fear of unwanted pregnancy without curtailing sexual relations became a critical plank in this platform. Married women wanted the opportunity to plan their families, which went hand in hand with designing their careers. Married, heterosexual women wanted the freedom to enjoy sex without fear of becoming solely dependent on their husbands for economic stability or intellectual stimulation.

The 1970s debates had not completely lost sight of these earlier concerns, linking poverty with birth control. Activist committees formed across the country to provide sex education, along with abortion counselling, and grassroots organizations formed to lobby the government to reform the laws. Women from the Saskatchewan-based Association for the Modernization of Canadian Abortion Laws, for example, started a radio talk show in 1966 to inform listeners about sex and birth control. They provided listeners with accounts of women who had called in desperation, hoping to secure some "magic potion" to alleviate the stress of an unwanted pregnancy. But, as they explained to the Regina *Leader Post*, "when you get calls like that [from desperate women], if you have any heart at all, you're fighting mad."[13] Emphasizing the humanitarian reasons for expanding legal abortion services, some reformers insisted that the current economic conditions demanded that women enter the workplace while at the same time offering few options in exchange that would relieve them of the burden of pregnancy or childcare. With growing expectations that they ought to participate in the economy, beyond their earlier working roles during wartime, women were no longer to be held hostage by biology. Middle-class women, increasingly expected to get jobs and hold down careers, now needed to plan their families and space out their children. If the 1920s birth controllers aimed their efforts at poor and working-class women whose large family sizes imperilled their mental and physical health, now middle-class women writing to commissioners on the Status of Women inquiry also clamoured for birth control to give "women control over their own bodies."[14]

Regardless of the legal prohibitions against advertising for birth control, let alone procuring abortions, pro-abortion groups like the Association for the Modernization of Canadian Abortion Laws gathered momentum across the country. They presented briefs to the government regarding the legalization of abortion, particularly in cases where a mother's or child's health was at risk, including for reasons of disability.[15] Those criteria, they argued, would not sufficiently address the problem of anxiety and risk associated with illegal abortions, but they recognized that a baseline was necessary for initiating legal reforms: "Even if those three points are included in the legislation, it won't solve the social problem. The majority of illegal abortions are not performed for these reasons."[16] The local press cited estimates of illegal abortions in Canada, ranging from 100,000 to 300,000, rates that did not even attempt to capture the number of cases referred to as "accidental miscarriages." While the article in the *Leader Post* made a strong case for decriminalizing abortion, and improving maternal health as a result, it ended with a statement from the association's president, Mrs Perron, reinforcing the view that the legal reforms were chiefly aimed at particular women: "Personally I feel a mature, intelligent woman should have the right to decide when she wants to have a child."[17] This view is reminiscent of older attitudes toward birth control and abortion that had been in circulation since the nineteenth century, namely that family planning was ultimately reserved for responsible, mature, morally upstanding, and intelligent citizens. Birth control, like population control, was something done *to* women, whereas family planning was something women could do themselves.

This conceptualization took on expanded meaning when applied to a global scale. Certain regions were cast as responsible for, or at least part of, the solution when they invested in birth control as a population-control measure. Making the matter one of international diplomacy, family planning was not just a women's issue but also one of global significance – one in which responsible westerners could participate: acting locally to improve conditions globally.

Press reports seized upon the notion of overpopulation as the main reason for reforming the laws. An article in the Saskatoon *Star Phoenix* pointed to what it considered successful policies in India and Japan to address the problem of population increase. Taking a global look, this article suggested that "many couples are too poor to afford, or too unintelligent to learn birth control methods. It [the genetic argument] says they are being allowed to overpopulate the world with offspring of inferior mental and physical competence." The article quickly moved on: "Agricultural economists say that this over-population is threatening to outstrip the world's food supply ... C.F. Bentley, dean of agriculture at the University of Alberta, had extended this reasoning into the area of world politics. He says that overpopulation increases poverty and that 'some poor country, under bad leadership, will ignite the third world war. Even small poor countries have the potential to

develop the end of civilization.'" Tying together the global burdens
of food distribution, environmental calamity, and political tyranny,
it seemed that birth control provided the solution to certain doom.
The article concluded with a clear message: "The law of this country has lagged behind accepted practice. The result borders upon
hypocrisy."[18] Indeed, Canada's position on birth control and abortion
lagged behind when considered in the context of global peacekeeping
efforts, particularly if one believed that those efforts depended on
stabilizing birthrates.

At the end of the 1960s, birth control had emerged as an important
solution to a growing – and frightening – list of world crises. Public
outcry over the conjoined issues of food supply and birthrates had
become more prevalent in the popular media.[19] Decades of political
uncertainty during the Cold War had sparked doubts about the capacity for political leaders to resolve ideological conflicts, and an emerging generation of restless youth looked to take matters into their
own hands.[20] Western nations, which had traditionally resisted birth
control, looked to a new era of embracing family planning as a feature
of economic planning and global security.

For federal civil servants, however, family planning was not solely
a feminist agenda, nor even a eugenics issue, but instead a matter of
managing the economy. The Family Allowance system had been in
place since 1945, as a component of the social reconstruction effort
in the postwar period. By the 1960s, the program had become a pillar
of the welfare state and part of the Canadian government's efforts to
reduce poverty and shape families. According to historian Raymond
Blake, the Canadian Tax Federation was quick to emphasize the
relationship between family size and poverty; "after all, the size of
the family was an important contributory factor to poverty."[21]

Over the 1960s, the Family Allowance program's responsibility for
addressing issues of poverty grew steadily. Civil servants debated
thresholds for financial support, whether based on income levels or
family size. For Quebec politicians, notably political leader René
Lévesque, who at the time was minister of family and welfare, the
issue remained one of jurisdiction. Income security, provincial autonomy, and health and welfare occupied a series of inquiries in the late
1960s and early 1970s, all of which were premised on the principle
that the Canadian family was the bedrock of the nation, and for
Lévesque, those decisions belonged within the provinces.

For many Canadians, however, the definition of family and marriage
entailed more than a set of government benefits, tax provisions, or

federally, or even provincially, defined categories. If civil servants were keen to plan an economy based on assumptions about the role of families, individual families too were increasingly participating in redefining the modern family. Some did so by testing common law provisions for living arrangements at tax time. Others lobbied for better divorce laws, custody provisions, or daycares for children of single mothers. According to Blake, the Economic Council of Canada reported in 1968 that "poverty in Canada was real, and noted that the number of poor were not in the thousands but, rather, millions." Antipoverty campaigns became part of a national strategy. Two years later, the Royal Commission on the Status of Women drew particular attention to the plight of single mothers, who disproportionately suffered from poverty.[22]

CANADIAN PARLIAMENTARY DEBATES

On 21 December 1969 the Canadian government finally amended its Criminal Code to decriminalize abortion, contraception, and some aspects of homosexuality. This change occurred only after a series of debates over the details of Bill C-150, which Parliament ultimately passed with a vote of 149 to 55. The vote had been preceded by three years of heated discussions over the terms of this multilayered and morally complicated law.

Trudeau had, as minister of justice in 1967, introduced the omnibus Bill C-150. The proposed amendments were complex. They targeted the Criminal Code of Canada, and taken together the changes represented 126 different elements. Hansard, the official records of the parliamentary debates, described the coalition of changes with this lengthy phrase: "Bill c-150, to amend the Criminal Code, the Parole Act, the Penitentiary Act, the Prisons and Reformatories Act, and to make certain consequential amendments to the Combines Investigation Act, the Customs Tariff and the National Defence Act, as reported ... from the Standing Committee on Justice and Legal Affairs." Discussions over how to tackle this sprawling proposal spilled over many sessions and many hours. The topic locked parliamentarians in debate and stimulated some anticipated contests over the moral and legal future of Canada's official position on sexuality and reproductive freedom.

Perhaps because the bill combined clauses on homosexuality with others on contraception and abortion, some members felt that the cumbersome nature of the bill was in fact a deliberate attempt to undermine Canadian family values. One Quebec Social Credit MP exclaimed of the proposed bill "that [it] is the height of irony. Never, as far as I know, during the last election campaign, has the present government or the Liberal party requested a free hand from the Canadian people to legalize homosexuality or abortion." One of his fellow caucus members, André-Gilles Fortin, put it more directly: "The passing of the omnibus bill on homosexuality will strike another blow, a fatal blow this time, at the Canadian family." Fortin maintained a conservative stance on the topic: "We ask ourselves whether by passing this bill, we will promote the progress of the Canadian family, or if we will not instead contribute to its disappearance, as was the case in socialist countries."[23] Earlier in his statement on the matter, Fortin had identified Czechoslovakia as one such socialist nation where the relaxation of policies on birth control and sexuality had allegedly corroded family values.[24] Conservative politicians worked to convince the country that only they could be trusted to protect Canadian families, setting in motion a political discourse that confused elements of conservatism with family values. Fortin explained that "if, under the pretext of safeguarding freedom, we prevent the Canadian family from growing we shall have committed a criminal act we will regret for the rest of our days."[25] Progressive Conservative MP Philip Rynard, a surgeon from Orillia, Ontario, complained,

> In Denmark and Sweden, there are new forms of marriage, social acceptance of homosexuality, abolition of censorship, permission to use soft drugs, compulsory sex education and easy access to contraceptives … It may be that when the limits of permissiveness are reached the Dutch, the Danes and the Swedes will find that they have not solved any of the age old moral problems but have simply transferred them to a different plane. Their experience has a certain fascination for the rest of the world, and they should not complain, as some of them do, when we curiously peer and prod.[26]

Without referring to fetal rights explicitly, one Quebec MP, René Matte, elaborated on the need to extend the liberal discourse to unborn children: "We must therefore recognize the full value of the child in his mother's womb, as well as his full right to life as a human being. Such is the freedom of the individual, which spreads over every instant of the life span, from the very beginning of the existence of a human being. Any human being has a right to be protected, even during his embryonary [*sic*] stage." He continued, "It is an awful thought that this may be the case in a Christian country. I wish to underscore the word 'Christian.'"[27] Moreover, Matte argued, "Are not 98 per cent of the population Christian? Is it a disgrace to put forward Christian principles? It is not. It is not scandalous to refer to them nor to say that the human being which is inside his mother's womb cannot protect himself, because he is not yet visible and to decide about his right to live. Mr Speaker, is that anti-Christian?" Rounding out his filibuster, Matte declared, "It would have been so simple, instead of taking so many precautions, not to legislate on abortion and homosexuality, and even if one did, to do so in a really adequate way, in a way that would promote the development of the country, instead of bringing about its decline."[28] Given the various pieces involved in this battery of amendments, much of the early debate focused on procedures and how to unpack the proposal to allow Parliament to sufficiently tackle the many implications of the proposed changes. Concerns touched on, predictably, religious interpretations of life and decency but also involved questions about the changes' effects on medical professionals. Would the law, for example, compel physicians to provide IUDs, or perform abortions, even if they personally objected to such procedures? Did the Canadian government have an obligation to protect the medical profession in this regard? Parliamentarians seemed more comfortable stepping into the shoes of physicians than those of fertile women when it came to discussing the nuanced features of power or available resources, as they determined who the law was for, and who it protected. One Member of Parliament remarked that "in Europe, I believe probably less than 4 per cent of abortions performed there are carried out for valid medical reasons. In the long run, the pressure of the affluent society, or of the just society—which, in effect means 'do what you want to do whether it is morally right or not' –may be great enough to break down the moral conscience of abortion committees and hospitals. This is what I fear."[29] In addition to concerns over how to protect medical professionals in the course of crafting the bill, some members worried that the bill ultimately protected wealthy Canadians in a move that introduced a slippery-slope argument to a broader degradation of morals.

This collusion of both local and global interests meant that decriminalizing birth control appealed across an unprecedented set of political and ideological lines. By the end of the 1960s, therefore, it seemed that amending the Canadian Criminal Code was something of a salutary gesture, a move that merely aligned emerging practices and attitudes with a law that appeared out of sync with modern life. Trudeau's motto, as it became known, seemed to fit neatly into this shifting landscape where the law stepped aside to allow citizens a greater opportunity to take their family planning into their own hands, aided by medical and scientific guidance. Manoeuvring into this new moral position on birth control also signalled a realignment with science as the preferred arbiter of sound public policy on the global scale.

Yet, despite this historical backdrop, the issues embedded in Canadian law were not obvious to everyone. Surprisingly, for Manitoba Conservative MP Walter Dinsdale, at least, the bill appeared to come out of nowhere: "I cannot understand why a government charged with the responsibility of leading this house and the nation is bringing in this change at this time when there has been no great public pressure or public clamor. The issue is seriously fraught with moral implications. We are bringing the morals and values of skid row into the salons and drawing rooms of the nation."[30] Much of Dinsdale's speech might have applied indiscriminately to different sections of the bill, but he elaborated as follows:

> We are concerned here with one of the most intimate and sensitive relationships between man and woman in human society. If we remove love from sex I suggest that we will destroy human personality ... What we are embracing is the *Playboy* philosophy ... Actually what we are embracing is the Mohammedan philosophy of hedonism. That is where the phrase, "The state has no business in the bedrooms of the nation," originated. The Arab attitude or Moslem [sic] attitude that as long as public decency is not debauched everything is alright ... In other words, what I don't see I should not and need not worry about.[31]

Dinsdale appears to have been playing into stereotypes in circulation at the time about the allegedly hypersexualized Arab male and the allegedly permissive, even hedonistic, culture of sexuality that fused misogyny with sexuality. Indeed, in 1968, American writer Joseph Rosenfeld published a titillating and rather lurid collection of stories and case studies from the "near east," which depicted Arab sexuality for American readers. His book, titled *The Orgiastic Near East*, seized upon this particular moment in history as concerns over sexuality and population control went global. Rosenfeld's book took those issues further, invoking elements of Arab misogyny as he painted an image of unchecked sexuality in non-Christian regions of the world. The book described westerners as prudish, secretive, and uncomfortable with sex, as opposed to the "Arab [who] has, as a rule, 'played up' the importance and incidence of things erotic, while his Western brother has only whispered about sexual activity."[32] These kinds of claims further underscored some of the ways that sexual liberation became part of an "othering" discourse, not the least of which pitted regions and religions against one another in terms of the moral upper hand.

Concerns over the decriminalization of abortions reinforced this perspective, while framing women as virtuous victims in need of protection. Dinsdale explained, "We are reversing completely values and traditions which have been the foundation stone upon which our western Christian civilization has been established." He went on to complain that "this is being done without any public pressure. The initiative has come from the government. There was a time when it was possible to say that all politicians were against sin and for motherhood. Here we have a reversal of this fundamental principle. Obviously ... we are downgrading the role of motherhood in this nation."[33] Though Dinsdale claimed to speak on behalf of western Christian ideals, he was not alone in speaking on behalf of religious communities.

Henry Latulippe, Quebec M P for the Social Credit Party of Canada, took the notion of divine rule one step further. He suggested that Canada was indeed quite different from many of the southern nations where population growth might pose an undue burden on resources. Instead, he explained, "Providence placed us in Canada and asked us to grow and multiply. The rules that are about to become law with regard to abortion cannot meet divine requirements. In Canada, the population should increase according to the views of Providence." Lest there be any confusion about how the nation should accomplish this growth, he added, "In Canada, the population is not large enough for the debts we have to pay. Instead of turning to massive immigration, we should protect our population, allow it to increase at the rate Providence would have it."[34] Latulippe's comments tapped into an undercurrent of pronatalism that continued to course through the debates as lawmakers attempted to balance traditions of nation building and nativism with the looming civil unrest, as women demanded equality, Red Power activists demanded recognition and retribution for cultural genocide, and Quebec sovereigntists engaged in a nation-building exercise of their own.

Within Parliament, representatives debated even the veracity of this issue among members of the public. Some, like MP and Ralliement des Créditistes leader Réal Caouette, stated that "the government is snowed under by thousands of letters from people protesting against Bill C-150." According to Caouette, this public reaction indicated that the government should retain strict laws. He acknowledged that Grace MacInnis, NDP MP, had claimed to be receiving letters in support of the changes to the bill, of which he had read ten.[35] He then said that if such letters existed they should be read in Parliament and the fact that they were not was proof enough to him that Canadians did not support the bill. Caouette was convinced by letters, petitions, and signatures that Canadians were against the bill and that his party was justified in delaying the vote with its filibustering tactics.

Despite the long-winded speeches about the divine order or natural birthrate and its relationship to healthy nation building, the discussions progressed and the Liberal Party held its ground in advancing Bill C-150. After getting past the definitions, and subdividing the discussion, the debate refocused in the remaining months on the criteria surrounding abortions. Even without religious opposition, the conditions for relaxing the law on abortion presented significant challenges, in large measure because it involved relying on physicians to carry out the procedure.

The bill came into effect in August 1969 but not without prolonged discussions about who would actually have the final say on the abortion issue. Even more so than with the Bill C-150's other categories, the abortion question descended into a debate over who would retain the ultimate legal responsibility, not over who might benefit from a relaxed abortion law or whose life might be most directly affected by having or not having access to abortion. As historian Beth Palmer has argued, the changes to the abortion laws paradoxically introduced a set of new barriers for women seeking abortions.[36] Namely, the new legislation mandated the therapeutic abortion committee, a board of "three doctors whose role was to determine whether the continuation of a pregnancy would impact on the physical or mental health of the woman."[37] The imposition of this review process created challenges for the timing of abortions. Assembling the TACs required coordinating schedules and personnel with the time-sensitive nature of abortions performed between eight and twelve weeks of pregnancy, as provinces went about setting upper limits of twelve weeks as the maximum allowable limit. Palmer suggests that the TACs also stimulated activists "to help women to access services through referrals, while others fought to further liberalize the laws ... [A]ctivists across the country used mock tribunals to put the laws on trial and hold the criminal system accountable."[38]

Requiring these TACs immediately raised concerns about the distribution of services, particularly in underserved communities. Eldon Woolliams, MP for Calgary North, pointed out that "under clause 18 of the bill a committee of doctors must be set up and the operation can only be performed in an accredited hospital if the doctors say that an abortion is necessary in their view to preserve the life and health of the mother." Placing control first and foremost in the hands of the doctors made it clear whose choice mattered most. Woolliams went on to criticize the proposal as being inherently discriminatory. However, his argument was not that it discriminated against women, per se, but rather that it made it very difficult for people living in rural communities to assemble the requisite committee in a timely manner to provide an abortion if requested. He stated that, "In remote parts of Canada far away from urban centres it is difficult or impossible to get a committee of doctors or to reach an accredited hospital. So this bill would be discriminating, by procedure only and not by law, against people living in these areas. For instance, Tisdale or Melfort, is 160 miles from Saskatoon where there are enough doctors and accredited hospitals."[39] Tisdale and Melfort might indeed struggle to assemble such committees, but Woolliams's emphasis pointed to deeper problems of discrimination in regions with even poorer access to medical services.

By the last month of the debate, the questions focused almost exclusively on the nature of the TACs and the distribution of services. Ultimately, the bill included the provision that "a qualified medical practitioner who procures the miscarriage of a female person, and a female person who permits a qualified medical practitioner to procure her miscarriage, would not ... be guilty of those offences if the therapeutic abortion committee of the hospital where the miscarriage was procured certified in writing, before the miscarriage was procured, that in its opinion the continuation of the pregnancy of the female person would or would be likely to endanger her life or health."[40]

As the bill reached its final reading, public resistance to its details mounted. The Victoria Abortion Reform Committee's Mrs S. d'Estrube pleaded with the government to take more aggressive steps toward liberalizing the clause on abortion, in particular, by removing the restriction to only those cases where a woman's physician agreed that continuing with the pregnancy would be detrimental to her health: "If you feel, as we do, that women should not have to bear babies which they do not want or cannot provide for – if you believe children should not be brought into an over populated world to suffer neglect and emotional deprivation – if you think our largely male Parliament has no business legislating a punitive 'morality,' of which women are frequently the scapegoats and innocent babies the victims – then we invite you to join us in our efforts."[41] D'Estrube's comments are revealing, in that they evoke established arguments for both population control and gender equality, a feature made clear in the drastic imbalance of gendered perspectives in Parliament. The disparity in the tenor of these conversations perhaps reflected deeper divisions that were not readily solved by simply changing the Criminal Code or declaring that the government was absolving itself of responsibility over the question of birth control. Shifting the power of choice to the medical profession and couching it in the protectionist language of health maintained a veneer of patriarchal authority. Meanwhile, women were busy reframing that discourse by highlighting family planning as a central feature of a vibrant and sustainable Canadian economy. Their discourse relied on equality, partnership, and choice, and they increasingly looked beyond the nation's border for inspiration.

THE WOMEN ARE COMING

Very shortly after the passing of the omnibus bill, in 1969, Canadian women began openly registering their frustration with the new law. The introduction of the TAC clause complicated the decision-making process, ensured delays in a procedure that relied on timely responses, and subjected pregnant women to what was in effect a morality trial before an assembly of physicians. Placing control in the hands of physicians undermined the philosophy of autonomy and choice that had animated contemporary feminist activism in the first place. Within weeks, women gathered in British Columbia as part of the Vancouver

Women's Caucus, to protest the bill and to march on Ottawa to demand further changes.[42] Their actions further underscored the near absence of women in Parliament. Indeed, during the 28th Parliament, in session from 1968 to 1972, Grace MacInnis, a New Democrat representing Vancouver (Kingsway), was the lone female representative. Her presence constituted 0.4 per cent, while male representation was 99.6 per cent.

As Canadian women gathered momentum and prepared to march on Ottawa – mirroring the 1935 On-to-Ottawa trek of unemployed men demanding work and wages – members of Parliament raised concerns with the prime minister. Ed Broadbent requested that someone in government should meet with the women protesting the abortion clause. Trudeau responded by suggesting that he was busy that day. The prime minister explained in Parliament that he had already met with women; he reiterated that the law had only recently been changed and that his government would not be exploring further amendments. He added that the women heading to Ottawa had not made an appointment, and therefore he could not be expected to meet with them: "They cannot just set a date themselves and expect us to meet them automatically."[43] In the event, it appeared that Trudeau had underestimated these women.

The timing was awkward. The Liberals had established the Royal Commission on the Status of Women in February 1967, only months before introducing the omnibus bill. The royal commission reported its findings on 7 December 1970, sixteen months after the bill came into effect. Whether deliberately or not, the views of women seemed to be omitted from the discussions surrounding abortion and birth control in the political sphere. Not to diminish MacInnis's participation in the parliamentary debates, but the lack of women's voices in these discussions became a rallying cry to bring women's issues into the public discourse. While the effectively exclusively male Parliament debated the proposed changes to laws on birth control and sexuality, the royal commission was conducting a cross-Canada survey and developing its own recommendations. The commission, led by CBC journalist Florence Bird, inquired into the equality of women in Canadian society, with an explicit focus on "critical issues for women [such as] poverty, family law, the Indian Act and the need for a federal representative for women."[44] Although the commission was not expressly tasked with determining the fate of birth control, the issue

predictably emerged in discussions about family, education, life expectancy, healthcare services, and women's roles in the economy. The
commission and the thousands of women who participated in its
hearings, presented briefs, or independently wrote to the commissioners recognized a clear link between birth control and their future role
as modern citizens.

At the core of the commission was an interrogation of women's
roles, from the view of men as well as women. From the opening
pages of its report, both women's relationship to family and the
implications of family planning are clear. It was paramount to the
commissioners not only that men's attitudes toward women change
but also that women embrace an ethos of liberation that allowed
them to make free and open choices about their futures, unencumbered
by expectations of performing particular roles and duties or through
the burden of their biology.

Much of the discussion focused on women's underacknowledged
abilities and their increasing opportunity to participate in the workforce,
due in no small measure to a declining birthrate. The report states,

> The fertility rate has been declining in Canada, as in many other
> western countries, owing to an increased use of birth control
> methods. In the middle of the last century, Canadian women
> who were still married at the age of 50 had borne an average
> of eight children. By the turn of the century the number had
> decreased to six, and, by 1961, to three, even before the wide
> spread use of the contraceptive pill. This means that the repro-
> ductive function no longer dictates the destiny of most women
> as it did in the past.[45]

The report explains how this represented a fundamental shift in
how women could and should plan their lives. With the advance of
new medical technologies designed specifically to improve women's
health, in areas of birth control as well as menopause, women were
having fewer children and living longer lives. This meant that they
had more opportunities to participate in the paid labour force and a
greater variety of options for education and careers than ever before.
Drawing on feminist writers from the United States, such as Gloria
Steinem, and the work of Parisienne scholar Simone de Beauvoir and
Belgian Suzanne Lilar, the commissioners considered local perspectives
from Canadian women and linked these local campaigns with an

international, intellectual movement that aimed to reframe women's lives through the language of choice and the science of planning. The report makes this point very clearly in a quote translated from Lilar's *Le malentuendu du deuxième sexe*: "With each passing day, the part of life ruled by biological factors becomes smaller, and that left to free choice, larger."[46]

The report examines the roots of stereotypes that had heretofore served to define modern women, showing how most of these images were informed by "Greek philosophy, Roman law, and Judeo-Christian theology—[which] have each held, almost axiomatically, that woman is inferior and subordinate to man and requires his domination." These assumptions, the commissioners suggest, were naturalized to the extent that they became part of the social order, when, in fact, "aside from physical differences, there has been no scientific proof of differences, either psychological or intellectual in the genetic inheritance of men and women." Therefore, the distinguishing feature is not borne out through either science or religion; instead, "women's child-bearing function and their physical differences have served as the basis for restrictive generalizations and overt discrimination."[47] Rejecting clichés that infantilize women as weaker, less intelligent, or less psychologically resilient, the commissioners tapped into emerging intellectual currents aimed at bringing scientific empiricism into harmony with civil rights activism. Much like the scientists seeking international expression for their theories of life sciences, evolutionary biology, and population control, the emerging feminism looked beyond national borders to build a political movement that relied on science to help overturn patriarchy. The commissioners also quoted anthropologist Margaret Mead, who "sees signs of a future in which there would be 'an emphasis on very small families and a high toleration of childless marriage ... parenthood would be limited to a smaller number of families ... adults who functioned as parents would be given special forms of protection.'" Mead also predicted, as quoted in the commission's report, that "limitations on freedom would be removed from women as a social group. Boys and girls would be differentiated not by sex-typed personality characteristics, but by temperament."[48]

The commissioners seized upon women's experiences around the globe to help challenge the local conditions that constrained women and men from generating the perspectives they needed to see beyond a patriarchal world view. Indeed, these broader perspectives were critical for establishing insight into local conditions. Women reported that in spite of the satisfaction they earned from joining the workforce, these feelings of accomplishment or even liberation from the traditional roles in the domestic sphere were soon replaced with guilt. The report makes the subtle point that "often a psychological conflict is an invisible barrier to freedom of choice for a woman."[49] Women were not the only ones struggling with this new outlook on gender roles. The report continues: "Many husbands are puzzled when their wives, to whom they feel they have given everything, develop interests of their own. This change in a husband's understanding of his wife's needs and aspirations will require him to make adjustments in his thinking about his own role as husband and father."[50] These comments relied on shifting psychological theories, coupled with ideas about sexuality, labour, and autonomy. The commission presented insights that went well beyond determining the fate of a particular policy or law, striking at the culture and psychology of western Judeo-Christian understandings of progress and justice. Changing those very long-standing traditions and conceptualizations was not a naïve enterprise but an essential step on a path of modernization.

Notably, planning and choice are threaded through the nearly five-hundred-page report. The underlying philosophical implication is clear: For women to be considered equal, as some sought, or to be valued as full citizens with different attributes, as others suggested, women had to be offered choices. This freedom of choice would not exist simply in relation to arguments about biology but filter into the workplace in strategic ways. Women had to be supported, psychologically and economically, to choose a career, whether inside or outside of marriage. Women had to have the opportunity to leave their home communities in search of advanced training with the full knowledge and security that they could succeed on their own. Women needed to be free to choose their partners based on their own criteria, not the spectre of pregnancy or fear of financial insecurity. In other words, women had to be remade as independent citizens with responsibility as well as freedom of choice.[51]

One immediate and practical recommendation focused on the Indian Act and the denial of rights afforded to women who risked losing their status for marrying "non-Indian" men. Pointing out the sexism in the laws that discriminated against women specifically, the commission expressed that "legislation should be enacted to repeal the sections of the [Indian] Act which discriminate on the basis of sex.

Indian women and men should enjoy the same rights and privileges in matters of marriage and property as other Canadians."[52] Further, the report recommends that Indigenous status also be granted to children, in an effort to reinstate rights that historically were removed from women and their children.

On the specific issue of birth control, the commissioners did not mince words: "The scientific control of the human reproductive function is one of the most important developments of this century."[53] The report goes on to refer to birth control as a feat of science in aid of gender equality, because it allows for planning to guide family formation: "Control of human reproduction has far-reaching consequences. It enables parents to plan the size of their families and the spacing of their children. It helps individuals and couples to reach a better sexual adjustment." And, to emphasize the point that science enabled this new political moment, the report continues by linking science to choice: "Like many forms of scientific progress, it [birth control] reduces the tyranny of natural forces over human beings; it makes possible more intelligent control of events; it increases personal freedom." The answer to this problem, according to the commissioners, is simple: "All this requires readjustments in the law, and reshaping of social customs and attitudes. Women, as the child-bearers, will be most affected by this new freedom and responsibility."[54] The report's authors were not blind, however, to some of the inherent inequities concerning the distribution of these medical technologies and the legacy of birth control as an instrument of control rather than choice. They acknowledged that, "in one sense, birth control is a social problem in Canada. Families with higher education and in higher income brackets have had easy access to birth control methods; the poor and less well-educated have not."[55]

After outlining the various birth control methods legally available, the report goes on to explain how the topic was psychologically and emotionally stressful because of the lack of services and information available to Canadian women. Despite the critical role of family planning in advancing gender relations and stabilizing the work force, the obstacles to birth control and sex education were reminiscent of older traditions and values that subscribed to an inferior view of women. The commissioners singled out the Roman Catholic Church and its views on nonprocreative sex, as confirmed in Pope John Paul's 1968 encyclical *Humanae Vitae*. Yet they also explained that Canada was, that year, home to over four million women of childbearing age, and the Toronto Family Planning Clinic, the largest such centre in Canada, had the capacity to respond to only 1,250 calls per year.[56] The report underscores the gross disparity between need and access, ultimately recommending "that birth control information be available to everyone" and "that the Department of National Health and Welfare (a) prepare and offer birth control information free of charge to provincial and territorial authorities, associations, organizations and individuals and (b) give financial assistance through National Health grants and National Welfare grants to train health and welfare workers in family planning techniques."[57] It goes on to suggest that the information and technology needed to be provided in remote regions as well as urban areas, reflecting the commission's understanding that the issue of birth control was a social problem.

As the commissioners astutely pointed out, sexual sterilization, although recognized as the most effective way to prevent pregnancy, had a reputation as a coercive surgery associated with eugenics. However, because of its effectiveness, commissioners recommended both clarifying its legal status as an operation and providing information through public health channels about sterilization as a birth control option. Indeed, as they noted, the procedure for men required only twenty minutes in a doctor's office, while for women it involved an overnight stay and a more invasive surgery. The commission advised that vasectomies should be considered within the range of public health options for family planning purposes. To that end, it also recommended "that the provinces and territories adopt legislation to authorize medical practitioners to perform non-therapeutic sterilization at the request of the patient free from any civil liabilities toward the patient or the spouse except liability for negligence."[58] With such improvements in birth control measures, the commissioners reasoned, the need for abortion might be eliminated altogether.

The issue of abortion struck at the heart of the philosophical divide between the commissioners and the parliamentarians who crafted the amendment on abortion. The creation of TACs, tasked with determining the relative health risk to the mother or fetus, left the choice in the hands of the medical establishment and made the mother vulnerable. According to the commission, "The principal benefactor of this law is the medical profession which will know exactly under what conditions a therapeutic abortion can be performed and criminal responsibility avoided."[59] In other words, women desperate to have an abortion but who either missed the window of opportunity or were turned down by a TAC might very well continue to explore options, leaving them vulnerable to increased health risks. Commissioners recognized this situation: "The current law cannot be relied upon to reduce the number of illegal abortions or the maternal deaths and injuries that follow the improper medical practices used in many illegal abortions."[60] The new law specified that a mother's life needed to be in grave danger before she could qualify for an abortion, a requirement that no doubt would have induced some women to take the risk of a non-medical abortion in an effort to procure relief from an unwanted pregnancy.

Surveys of Canadian women, as well as women living in the United States and Europe, routinely indicated that the majority of medical abortion requests came from married women who already had children. In Czechoslovakia, for example, 82 per cent of abortions performed legally in 1962 were for married women. The effective decriminalization of abortion in Czechoslovakia had drastically reduced reliance on illegal and more risky abortions. Alfred Kinsey's research in the United States had a smaller sample size but concurred with this research.[61] The commissioners had asked Canadian women about their own experiences procuring abortions and found that 43 per cent of respondents favoured an abortion-on-demand approach, within the first trimester. According to the commission's report, respondents to a *Chatelaine* magazine poll voiced an even higher degree of support: over 50 per cent of those polled in both French and English favoured an abortion-upon-request model.[62] Overwhelmingly, the commission's recommendations aligned with the standard of individual choice and personal control. The commissioners acknowledged too that, despite the sententious rhetoric, whether political or religious, most individuals, regardless of their faith or politics, supported a model that reinforced the philosophical principle of autonomy and choice.

CONCLUSION

Despite the early rhetoric about the "population bomb" and the environmental calamities that overpopulation would trigger, Canadians for the most part looked inward in this moment. Legal debates in Parliament invoked international trends in a superficial attempt to galvanize support for timely action. MP Grace MacInnis played an important role, but the parliamentary discussions were overwhelmingly dominated by men, who tended to frame the debate as one of national significance for what it revealed about Canada as a Christian nation. In contrast, thousands of women participated in the Royal Commission on the Status of Women. In this context, they readily looked beyond the national borders to link their feminist movement with a broader geographical and historical set of struggles against patriarchal institutions and practices that made women captive to biology. Yet here, too, Canadian feminists tended to look to other westerners for insight into a modern feminism that conceptualized reproductive choice as largely a prerogative of white, heterosexual women. The idea of linking arms with the poor mothers of India, for example, did not come through explicitly in the campaigns for feminist sisterhood.

While the tenor of these debates borrowed elements from the global conversation on population control, the conversation was anything but consistent and coherent when it came to charting a path for Canadian families. The disconnect between the parliamentary debates and the royal commission suggests that the notion of birth control featured very differently in these public forums, while the ties to global struggles were more abstract than concrete justifications for altering Canadian encounters with birth control or abortion. These contradictions continued to complicate the moral ground on birth control distribution as Canadians faced decisions in their own homes or communities. Healthcare administrators and civil servants took matters into their own hands when it came time to apply the new laws and to convince Canadians to adjust their values regarding who should embrace birth control as a modern liberal subject.

CHAPTER TWO

Politics of Health in the Global North

On 1 April 1973, CBC Television's national Sunday news program, *Weekend*, led with a sensational story of the involuntary sterilization of Indigenous women. Reporter Charlotte Gobeil interviewed women from two Mackenzie Valley communities who said they were sterilized without their knowledge or consent at the federal government's Charles Camsell Hospital in Edmonton. The reporter also heard from a missionary and community activists who implied that the sterilizations were part of a government effort to limit the growth of northern Indigenous populations. Not surprisingly, the CBC program prompted questions in the House of Commons, which triggered a frantic bureaucratic effort to refute the charges. Within a week, health minister Marc Lalonde sent a sharply worded denial to CBC president Laurent Picard that was simultaneously released to the press. The minister charged that the public broadcaster had its facts wrong – the women had indeed signed consent forms, claimed Lalonde – and had exploited the "Indian people" for the sake of sensationalism. Lalonde vehemently denied the program's suggestion that the government was "pursuing a deliberate program to sterilize native women in Canada."[1]

It was not the first time that controversy surrounded the federal government's role in supplying contraceptive services for Indigenous people, and it would not be the last. But this particular episode exposed the contentious politics of reproduction in the post-1969 era. While the 1969 amendments to the Criminal Code had liberalized Canadians' access to birth control, including contraceptives and abortion, and the government had assured Canadians that the state had no business in their bedrooms, bureaucratic surveillance of, particularly, Indigenous women's reproduction increased. At the same time, in the wake of the government's disastrous 1969 White Paper, which proposed the termination of its treaty and customary commitments, resurgent Indigenous political organizations increasingly viewed the state as intent on what Harold Cardinal termed "cultural genocide."[2] Cardinal was a young Indigenous leader who in 1968, at the age of twenty-three, was already leading the Indian Association for Alberta and who famously challenged not only Prime Minister Trudeau's White Paper but also, later, Trudeau's "Just Society," which Cardinal cleverly reframed in his book *The Unjust Society*. An emerging spokesperson for and recognized leader of Indigenous people in Canada, Cardinal put Indigenous issues in the spotlight with his challenge to the federal government. Moreover, igniting claims of cultural genocide invoked family planning and charged the federal government with extinguishing Indigenous people from the Canadian mosaic.

This chapter examines the shifting meanings of contraceptive technologies for women seeking reproductive autonomy while acknowledging that the terms and conditions on which Indigenous women accessed these technologies were rarely of their own making. Longstanding tensions related to race, gender, and place continued to complicate the issue of reproductive rights.[3] We argue that in spite of the federal government's claims to be pulling itself out of Canadian bedrooms, for Indigenous women the state became more invested in their reproductive bodies than ever before.[4] Women responded, unsurprisingly, in diverse ways, sometimes embracing the new reproductive health services and other times rejecting these new technologies that some viewed as a further attempt to control Indigenous populations.

Our study closely examines the federal government's response to shifting cultural ideas about reproductive health services at a historic moment when feminists and sovereigntists activated the political discourse with the language of fertility and population control, albeit with very different motivations. In the 1970s, these debates were impregnated with new cultural meaning in the wake of the decriminalization of contraception and abortion, ushering in a technology that promised women autonomy over their reproductive bodies. But those same services also clashed with the language of sovereignty and population control, whether among Quebec nationalists or Red Power activists, who articulated resistance toward contraception as a form of population control.

Canada's North became a testing ground for competing interpretations of population control. Some Canadian scholars have claimed that eugenics programs across the country disproportionately targeted First Nations and Métis people, and the government stretched those programs northward in the 1970s in a less formalized program of neo-eugenics. For example, Yvonne Boyer reports that Indigenous people were considered part of the "wrong" social group. She further suggests that residential schools might have been involved in sterilizing First Nations students in western and northern Canada.[5] Similarly, Paul Primeau argues that a statistical bias toward sterilizing Indigenous people existed in the Alberta eugenics program. He combines this programmatic evidence with other historically sensitive studies of childbirth, hospitalization, and colonialism to illustrate how concepts of race commingled with presumptions about intelligence and mental hygiene, which systematically brought Indigenous people under state surveillance.[6] More recently, Karen Stote has argued that Indigenous women "were the most prominent victims of the [eugenics] board's attention" and suggests that "those in Canada most likely to fit this categorization [of feeblemindedness] and on whom Alberta's legislation was disproportionately applied were Aboriginal peoples; more specifically young Aboriginal women."[7] Stote selectively examines the federal government's Indian Health Services records, which she says reveal that the Canadian government engaged in coercive sterilizations amounting to a genocide in the late 1960s and 1970s in the Northwest Territories.[8]

This literature identifies Indigenous women as victims within an extended practice of eugenics or population control that targeted certain women on the basis of race; however, it overlooks the possibility that some of these women sought access to birth control technologies, including voluntary sterilization. Federal health bureaucrats struggled to balance the need to provide services to communities in the northern territories with the need to minimize expenses. The issue of contraception created new complications for IHS bureaucrats, who attempted to comply with the new federal laws but remained wary of birth control's recent association with eugenics and forced sterilization abuses. They ultimately defended their decisions to make contraception available, particularly as it reduced maternal and infant-mortality rates, but they encountered difficulties in distributing clear information. For example, IHS bureaucrats asked a group of Inuit women of "above average education for the eastern Arctic" to translate a sterilization consent form written in Inuktitut syllabics. Of the nine women consulted, two thought it meant to have an abortion, five thought it meant to have an operation and have no more babies, and two had difficulty determining what the consent form was for. As one bureaucrat put it, "under the circumstances it would seem that the form needs a bit of re-drafting to ensure that people are fully aware of what they are agreeing to."9 This anecdote indicates that the distribution of birth control in the 1970s cannot be neatly described as either uniformly coercive or unilaterally requested. These conventional divisions of coercion and choice do not sufficiently capture the range of experiences faced by women living north of the sixtieth parallel, for whom reproductive health services remained limited and whose bodies were also politicized in contemporary political movements activated by the language of sovereignty – movements that cherished women's reproductive roles and emphasized pronatalism as an essential ingredient in self-determination.

Women living in these communities, however, responded to reproductive health services in diverse ways, revealing some of the gendered contours of these national and international debates over choice and sovereignty in the 1970s. By mid-decade the issue of contraception in the North had gained national publicity, as the federal government was accused of coercively sterilizing women. However, women in one community of approximately three hundred people in the eastern Arctic wrote to the federal health minister to counter the claims of genocide:

> We the ... Public Health Committee are going to write our minds regarding sterilization. We hear a lot about sterilization. We believe that sterilization should not be judged purely on moral reasons. There are people like us here in ... [Nunavut] who have had such operations done to them so we know the doctors do not perform operations on people without making sure that the person understands what they are being operated for. In this case the doctors do not decide whether to sterilize a person or not. There are those who especially ask for it. There are those who need it but if they do not want it they cannot be operated on. Those people who are talking now on the radios regarding sterilization are saying that the doctors perform sterilizations on people without telling them that they are getting sterilized. We think that those statements are false, because the doctors can operate only after consulting with the patient.10

These women's voices encourage us to tease apart the layers of morality and rhetoric to appreciate the complex nature of reproductive politics at this time.

Widening the focus beyond Canada's borders helps to draw other interpretations into the equation, allowing us to place the loosely defined Canadian North in the global context of population control. American feminist scholar Laura Briggs published a revealing study in 1998 where she examined the discourses of "forced sterilization" in Puerto Rico. Though overwhelmingly Catholic, Puerto Rico was one of the testing sites for the birth control pill and has a long and complicated colonial relationship with the United States. Briggs followed the lead of other American feminists who describe Puerto Rican women as victims of a vicious US foreign policy that had used them for experiments and also facilitated sterilization surgeries in accordance with eugenics theories. Over the course of her work, Briggs conducted oral interviews and uncovered a local feminist movement that challenged this conceptualization. She found women who had requested sterilizations in spite of their Catholicism, poverty, and race. In other words, she found women who acted remarkably similar to American middle-class women. The problem, Briggs explains, was that "mainland feminism engaged in what [Gayatri Chakravorty] Spivak has shown us is the problem of speaking on behalf of the subaltern, forcing a narrative from the bodies of poor Puerto Rican women in order to authorize its own politics."[11] The resulting historical interpretation, she contends, inaccurately aligns Puerto Rican feminism with "nationalism and pronatalism in Puerto Rico [that] had historically been associated with conservative Catholicism, the right wing, and antifeminism."[12]

Canadian Indigenous women's activism and feminism grew in the late 1960s, at times in solidarity with other women's organizations and feminists. A common focus was the gender discrimination provisions in the Indian Act where Indigenous women (and their children) lost their "Indian" status upon marriage to a non-Indigenous man.[13] Court challenges based in the discourse of human and civil rights and gender equity continued throughout the 1970s until the Indian Act was finally amended in 1985.[14] But these efforts also directly challenged claims by the nascent National Indian Brotherhood, made in response to the 1969 White Paper proposals, that the Indian Act, despite its oppressive colonialist agenda, was the sole recognition of the unique legal status of Canada's "Indians." To amend the Indian Act was to threaten band governance and the only means available to exercise what Cardinal termed their "sacred rights" as sovereigns.[15] Cast as selfish individualists and "women's libbers," the women's fight for reforms was dismissed at the time by the Indian Brotherhood as anti-Indian, inauthentic, and indeed dangerous to Indigenous sovereignty and self-government.[16]

If Indigenous activists created fraught relationships with Indigenous leadership by organizing their advocacy efforts around individual rights and gender equality, they also found themselves marginalized within the larger liberal feminist movement. What Joyce Green calls the "unthinking racism" of the white, middle-class women's movement erased the economic and political oppressions that Indigenous women faced.[17] Writing in 1989 in a major Canadian feminist journal, Kanien'kehá:ka (Mohawk) activists articulated an explicitly Indigenous women's movement that was critical of both liberal feminism and male-dominated Indigenous leadership. Drawing on their own cultural teachings as well as broader transnational Indigenous critiques of colonialism, the activist and writer Skonaganleh:rá noted,

> I understand the nature of being defined as a "feminist," and wanting some sense of equality, but frankly, I don't want equality. I want to go back to where women, in aboriginal communities … were treated as more than equal – where man was helper and woman was the centre of that environment, that community. I suppose equality is a nice thing and while I suppose we can never go back all the way, I want to make an effort at going back to at least respecting the role that women played in communities.[18]

Scholar Mary Ellen Turpel built on these foundations to advocate for a social, economic, and political renaissance to counter the colonialism – "patriarchy and paternalism" – of the Canadian state and society that ravaged both First Nations women and men, stating, "I have found that it is difficult for white feminists to accept that patriarchy is not universal."[19]

Historically contingent and rooted in the swirling identity politics of liberal feminism, sovereignty, and self-government, a parallel, though separate, theoretical stance emerged that celebrated Indigenous women's "traditional" and maternalist roles. Based on interviews with activist women, Grace Ouellette theorized that Indigenous women inhabit a "fourth world," different from mainstream feminism, where a "unique worldview underlies their actions and strategies."[20] Framed around a Circle of Life (or Medicine Wheel) philosophy where everything has its own place and meaning in nature, women's role as nurturers, caregivers, and child-bearers is taken as a natural phenomenon and not – as many non-Indigenous feminists see it – a social construction.[21] Ouellette's research suggests that Indigenous women perceived their multiple oppressions in colonialist policies, rather than solely at the hands of patriarchy, and tended to eschew the term "feminism."

Maternalism and motherhood are inherent in a transnational Indigenous reform strategy that invokes "motherwork," or women's unique role in procreation and the nurturing of children and communities. As Indigenous activism it appeals to traditions of "responsibilities" and a holistic sense of power, as opposed to the rights-based power that western feminists express. As American scholar Lisa Udel explains, "In order to do motherwork well, Native women argue, women must have power."[22] Maternalism as a political stance emerged in part in reaction to colonial experiences that degraded Indigenous motherhood generally and, in the US context, by the sterilization abuses in the mid-1970s that physically removed the capacity to fulfill this function of mothering.[23] But motherwork in the fourth world would also include regaining the sexual and reproductive autonomy that was suppressed by the imposition of Christian capitalism.[24] These institutional barriers to motherhood fused elements of patriarchy with colonial and evangelical legacies that had created a different set of dynamics for Indigenous women negotiating their place in the modernizing rights discourse.

At the same time, a small school of Indigenous feminism provides a more explicit critique of colonialism's gendered power relations.[25] It shows how Indigenous women and their communities are directly affected by racism and sexism and examines oppression in colonial as well as Indigenous governance. As Green recounts, in the 1970s Indigenous feminists "educated" western feminists who were "unfamiliar" with issues of colonialism, racism, and sexism.[26] But they also deployed their feminism carefully and differently.[27] This plurality of Indigenous feminisms is also conceptualized as an analytical "tool" rather than "identity politics" in a broad effort to achieve gender justice, underscoring the need to appreciate the fluidity of Indigenous feminisms.[28]

In the case of sterilization records in the Northwest Territories, and their historical examination, the politics of motherhood provides an important analytical corrective. While federal health bureaucrats pointed to improvements in maternal and infant mortality as proof that colonial control of Inuit birthing improved health, Inuit women organized to return childbirth to their communities. Pauktuutit (Inuit Women's Association) prioritized and politicized the revival of traditional midwifery as essential to cultural survival.[29] The loss of control over childbirth became a "metaphor for the loss of political control," shifting from being solely a women's issue to inform the larger Inuit political agenda of self-government.[30]

Women living north of the sixtieth parallel bore witness to these kinds of debates without necessarily having recourse to many of the provincial organizations or health services available to their southern Canadian counterparts. Canada's territories, in these debates, took shape as a region under federal control, requiring health services that mirrored provincial provisions; however, as Mary Jane McCallum notes, public health services in the territories had languished in scope, accessibility, staffing, and resources.[31] The regional and jurisdictional differences were further complicated by cultural and medical assumptions about Inuit and First Nations populations and their desire to control fertility. As the federal government looked northward to expand health services, it encountered a more diverse set of reactions than officials had anticipated. The issue of providing reproductive healthcare services in the North moved well beyond a matter of jurisdiction; instead, it embroiled federal civil servants in a much more contested matter of neocolonial population control. As the debate shifted from one of service provision to birth control for Indigenous women, the regional contours also drifted southward, enveloping provincial communities and reframing the issue as one of Indigenous reproduction, contraception, feminism, and population control. Health bureaucrats, meanwhile, struggled to find a consistent foothold in the changing rights discourse without sufficiently appreciating how women in the North experienced this cultural-medical shift in reproductive health services.

HEALTHCARE SERVICES
IN THE PROVINCIAL NORTH

In the early 1950s, incidents of surgical sterilization at Miller Bay Indian Hospital near Prince Rupert, BC, came to the attention of Indian

Health Service bureaucrats in Ottawa.[32] British Columbia and Alberta had passed sexual sterilization acts in 1933 and 1928, respectively, and established eugenics boards to recommend and adjudicate decisions for these operations. In British Columbia, the eugenics board was ostensibly created to help reduce the costs of maintaining people in expensive state-run institutions, when they could be cared for in the community after reducing the risk of procreation.[33] The so-called Indian hospitals fell within federal jurisdiction and therefore were not subject to routine assessments by the provincial eugenics board members, but the practice of sterilization did not cleave neatly to these jurisdictional distinctions.[34]

Near Prince Rupert, Miller Bay was one of twenty-two federally owned and operated Indian hospitals established in Canada during and after World War II. A redundant military installation initially repurposed to isolate and treat tuberculosis among Indigenous people, Miller Bay, like the other Indian hospitals, quickly emerged as a general hospital treating all conditions based on race, not disease. Indigenous communities, regularly excluded from local hospitals and left without treatment, welcomed the 1946 opening of Miller Bay Indian Hospital.[35] The influx of wartime American and Canadian military personnel had disrupted Indigenous communities throughout the Northwest in a number of ways, including severe epidemics of infectious disease that followed the building of the Alaska Highway and the Canol Pipeline.[36] But it was the government's larger colonializing project to isolate Indigenous people in the interests of settler society that prompted its extension of medical services.

In 1954, Dr G.R. Howell, the Miller Bay hospital's medical superintendent, solicited input from his superiors regarding the legality of sexually sterilizing women: "A few of our patients have asked us whether they could have this operation during the past year and it has been performed on three of them. We are however most anxious to protect ourselves in every way and to know the law on the subject. I would greatly appreciate a legal opinion."[37] Howell's use of the passive "it has been performed" would suggest that he did not perform the surgeries. The doctor, a former sanatorium patient himself whose health was deteriorating, spent much of his time at home in Prince Rupert, leaving care of the 175 patients to three staff officers at the hospital – one of whom was "not licensed to practice medicine and probably will not be able to obtain a license," according to a departmental inspector.[38] Howell's disturbingly belated request for direction caused concern in both the regional and national IHS offices. His superiors assured themselves that the women's health status must surely have necessitated the surgery and that Howell must have observed all ethical, medical, and surgical considerations. Nevertheless, IHS director Dr Percy Moore claimed to know nothing of the legal implications of surgical sterilization, though he believed such procedures were subject to provincial authority. He directed the departmental solicitor to look into the matter generally, as well as specifically with respect to British Columbia.[39]

Alberta's eugenics program had encountered similar challenges when confronted with cases of men and women from reserves. Indeed, within the context of the most open and aggressive eugenics program in Canada, concerns about sterilizing "Indians" produced considerable debate among program architects and Indian agents. Regarding a case in 1937, an agent engaged with both provincial and federal authorities in determining how to proceed:

The [Indian Affairs] Department has no power to authorize the sterilization of an insane Indian. It has no objections to the operation and would regard it with approval if carried out in accordance with the laws and regulations of the Province. It cannot, however, agree that any Indian should be sterilized without the consent of his relatives, and of himself as well, if he is mentally competent to understand the results of the operation. It is not beyond the realm of possibility that Indians might get the impression that there was a conspiracy for the elimination of the race by this means.[40]

The Indian agent later stressed that the operation should be deferred until the provincial eugenics board had obtained consent from the patient's family. Under the guidelines of Alberta's Sexual Sterilization Act, patients with sufficiently low intelligence quotients were not required to give consent, meaning that patients could legally be sterilized without their knowledge or consent.[41] In this case the provincial authorities responded to the IHS, claiming that "the patient is not willing to be sterilized but, according to the present Alberta Sterilization Act, his consent would not be necessary. Notwithstanding this latter fact it has not been our policy to operate where there are extenuating circumstances, which, in this case, would be the fact that he is an Indian."[42]

Sexual sterilization, difficult to access by putatively normal women and men, was wielded by eugenics boards to protect the province from the progeny of the so-called mental defectives and the "feeble-minded."[43] Nevertheless, the surgery, whether for health or purely eugenic concerns, required patients (or their guardians, or the provincial secretary) to provide written consent for treatment. Director Moore hoped the department's blanket form that patients signed upon admission to hospital might be amended to fit the special circumstances of voluntary sterilization. Indeed, "Form 7819: Application for Medical Treatment" concerned itself with limiting who might access IHS treatment while also limiting the services that might be provided. Moreover, upon admission, patients were required to consent to any and all treatment, presented on the form as follows: "I authorize to be performed on my person whatever examination, treatment or operation is indicated in the opinion of the medical authorities and I undertake to co-operate fully in all measures to maintain treatment and discipline."[44] The broadly coercive nature of the consent form did not meet the needs of voluntary sterilization, so department solicitor J.C. Hanson sought direction from British Columbia's provincial secretary in interpreting the Sexual Sterilization Act. As Hanson noted, the provincial act allowed that "an operation for sterilization may be performed by certain persons provided that a consent is obtained in writing from various parties."[45] Legal advisers determined that surgical sterilization could be performed only if further childbearing would endanger the life of the mother or adversely affect her health. But, Dr Moore remained concerned about the circumstances that would determine the necessary medical grounds for the procedure: Who would decide?[46] Ultimately, he settled on a policy whereby the patient required separate examinations by at least two physicians who then submitted in writing their reasons for recommending the procedure; written consent of both the patient and her spouse was also required. It seems clear that through negotiation with their doctors, these few women at Miller Bay gained access, albeit briefly, to a reproductive technology that allowed them to control their fertility.

Medical anthropologists and social workers have attempted to bring to light some of the experiences of First Nations and Inuit people through ethnographic research. For example, in the 1980s anthropologist John D. O'Neil revealed a number of cases, primarily of women, who were sterilized without their knowledge or consent in the 1960s and 1970s. One woman recalled, "The only other time I was sad like this was when I found out I couldn't have any more children. They did a hysterectomy in Churchill [Manitoba], but I didn't know about it. I am still angry about that."[47] These operations often coincided with treatment for other complaints, from depression to tuberculosis or cancer, and were not explained to the women by the physicians who performed the surgeries. In oral histories on the experience of being evacuated from their communities for childbirth, Inuit women complained about being separated from their community and about the loss of control over the ways they gave birth. As Patricia Kaufert and John O'Neil argue, this "colonial penetration" in the Arctic shifted the impact of resettlement, poverty, and disease "to the body of the Inuit woman."[48] Seeking and obtaining health services at all seemed to coincide with unsolicited reproductive healthcare interventions by a system that continued to operate under eugenic laws both where they existed and where they did not.

But the issue of sterilization and birth control was not always straightforward or uniformly applied. Throughout 1955 the IHS had received orders from Miller Bay for supplies that "could not be interpreted otherwise than as contraceptives."[49] Bureaucrats were concerned that an unrestricted supply of contraceptives provided through public funds might raise questions about IHS policy, not least since the practice was illegal (and would remain so for another thirteen years).[50] This inherent paradox reinforces the importance of race and region in reproductive health services: contraception remained illegal, and requesting it connoted a degree of criminal behaviour, while laws and medical professionals continued to justify coercive sterilization on the basis of its protective benefits for society as a whole. Indigenous women seeking birth control, much like their non-Indigenous counterparts, were rebuffed as immoral actors while eugenics board members claimed the moral upper hand in sterilizing people who were expected to be a drain on society. As the Ontario Medical Association (OMA) maintained at that time, "voluntary sterilization of the healthy should never be done."[51]

But, as McLaren and McLaren argue, many Canadians, including several physicians, had since the 1940s increasingly embraced both the practice of birth control and its advocacy once they understood how it might most usefully control the reproduction of "welfare cases" and other marginalized groups.[52] Physician-bureaucrats at IHS understood that they need only claim that the contraceptives would be considered necessary as life-saving procedures to protect themselves and their colleagues from any legal liability. In the director's reasoning, "It is my opinion that in certain circumstances prevention of conception may prolong life. I believe that the opinion is open to argument depending on religious background and training." Moore explained that IHS would provide contraceptive materials and individual medical officers and contracting physicians would be free to prescribe them as they saw fit: "It is assumed that a qualified practitioner knows what he is about, conforms both with the accepted teachings of his school and the accepted practice in the province in which he resides, and shall at all times attach due importance to the religious beliefs of the individual." Moore claimed that his policy of having no policy also upheld the "cardinal rule" of IHS: "not to interfere between a physician and his patient."[53] His latter claim was more than a little misleading since IHS regularly refused to authorize (and therefore fund) services or procedures that it deemed unnecessary or costly.[54] Nevertheless, IHS fully embraced the opportunity to provide birth control, in keeping with many socially conservative institutions – including the medical and legal professions and social welfare agencies – that, as historian Brenda Appleby argues, increasingly accepted the utility of contraception to mitigate class and racial tensions while preserving their privileged social positions.[55]

With the development of oral contraceptives, and Canada's Food and Drug Directorate's 1961 approval of "the Pill" for therapeutic use, women had access (through an accommodating physician) to nearly 100 per cent effective birth control that did not require the cooperation of their male partners. When, a year later, accounts from drugstores for prescriptions for Indigenous women began appearing on the IHS regional superintendent's desk in Edmonton, Dr W.L. Falconer refused to compensate the druggists. Citing "controversy on the use of this drug and probably some detrimental effects," Falconer advised that nurses should not distribute contraceptives; instead, physicians should be required to complete a special-treatment form indicating medical necessity. Only once the required paperwork was complete would IHS provide the pills from its own stocks. To this, Moore added a handwritten note: "I don't think this is a good directive."[56]

Indeed, less than a month later Moore informed all regional superintendents that "the hormone preparation Enovid" was available through IHS stocks and "supplies have been sent to quite a few field establishments on requisition." He did warn that "in view of the great hew [sic] and cry that resulted from the Thalidomide episode," physicians should understand the "possible toxic reactions."[57] Of particular concern was thromboembolic disease, or the formation of blood clots in the veins, a warning issued in August 1962 by Ortho Pharmaceuticals regarding its progestin-estrogen preparation, Ortho-Novum Tablets.[58] It appears IHS chose to stock Searle's Enovid (which posed the same health risk) because it was marginally cheaper, at $824.50 for 10,000 tablets packaged in 120-tablet bottles, compared with $976.78 for Ortho-Novum.[59] Moore considered that the reports of a connection between thromboembolic disease and oral contraceptive use might indeed be describing a coincidence; nevertheless, he suggested that Enovid should not be "given out by the nurses alone" but be issued by or on the order of a medical officer, that the drug should not be given to women living in remote areas infrequently visited by a field nurse, and that nurses should be reminded of the common symptoms of phlebitis (inflammation of a vein).[60]

It is clear that contraceptive information and technologies were made available to physicians and their Indigenous patients, but what is less clear is how and why healthcare workers promoted the technologies and how that information was received. That both Moore and Falconer before him felt compelled to warn specifically against the distribution of oral contraceptives by field nurses may indeed point to a widespread practice. Women, particularly in smaller communities with nursing stations, were far more likely to receive medical services and advice from nurses than from physicians; moreover, women may have been more likely to discuss very personal details about their reproductive health with another woman. In northern British Columbia, nurses continued to dispense oral contraceptives "if the husband and the priest are in agreement."[61] Nevertheless, as a reversible form of contraception, where women could choose whether to continue taking the prescription, birth control pills may have provided some measure of reproductive autonomy.[62]

In 1963, A.R. Kaufman – a rubber manufacturer and birth control advocate whose Kitchener, Ontario, Parents' Information Bureau (PIB) had provided contraceptives and surgical sterilization for the working classes since the Depression – offered to provide IHS with free birth control advice and supplies to manage the "tragic conditions ... aggravated by pathetic overcrowding due to high birth rates" in Inuit villages. Recommending surgical sterilization for Inuit men, Kaufman made clear his continued interest in eugenics: "Welfare work without family limitation is not going to be sufficient. Three generations of reliefees [sic] in one family should be convincing evidence for those who wish to consider the problem impartially." IHS director

Moore thanked Kaufman for his interest and assured him that "any Eskimo who requests information regarding birth control is provided with same by our doctors who are at liberty to order contraceptive drugs if it is in the interest of the patient or the family."[63] But in the 1960s, birth control took on far wider dimensions as "population control" where uncontrolled fertility came to be most closely associated with the poor and racialized in Canada and abroad.

CANADA'S NORTH GOES SOUTH

In the aftermath of World War II, a neo-Malthusian spectre of "population explosion" in the Third World captured the attention of many who saw unchecked fertility as both an economic and a Cold War geopolitical threat.[64] A transnational network of public and private interests including the American-funded and -controlled Population Council and International Planned Parenthood Federation emerged in the 1950s and 1960s to identify and meet the threat of overpopulation.[65] Population-control movements had in common the tendency to characterize social and political problems as pathologies with a biological basis; people in the postwar decolonizing world were viewed not as individuals but rather as populations that could be shaped by science and politics.[66] Population control became associated with progressive campaigns to alleviate poverty, which fused race and economic status together as the politics of region faded from the picture. The language of population control in the Global South emphasized a strain on resources and overpopulation, features that did not resonate in the Canadian North. The federal government's reaction reveals that population control in Canada had more to do with managing its Indigenous citizens than with concerns for overcrowded regions.

With its legal prohibitions against birth control at home, Canada was forced to abstain from a 1962 United Nations vote to support contraception use in the Third World.[67] But British expats George and Barbara Cadbury worked to claim a Canadian voice the next year by founding the Canadian Federation of Societies for Population Planning, an alliance of birth control societies that subsequently joined the IPPF.[68] The federation later changed its name to the less explicit Family Planning Federation of Canada (FPFC), and George Cadbury became director of the IPPF.[69] In 1963, Robert Prittie, NDP MP and an executive member of the FPFC, introduced Bill C-64, the first private member's bill calling for the decriminalization of birth control. Structured like the IPPF with formal decentralization, the Family Planning Federation of Canada included a range of advocates, from women's rights groups to population planning groups, and like the IPPF, its informal coordination by key leaders such as the Cadburys kept the ostensibly independent groups headed in the same direction.[70] The FPFC's brief to the House of Commons Standing Committee considering changes to the Criminal Code outlined four objectives: the first was to "encourage good citizenship through responsible family life," while the other three were all concerned with limiting population growth, including aiding international population-control efforts.[71] Enjoying a postwar economic and baby boom, Canadians across the political spectrum increasingly accorded the freedom of "responsible parenthood" to the middle and upper classes. The poor (globally and locally) continued to produce the wrong kinds of families with far too many children because women either would not or could not control their fertility. ·

Borrowing the language of US President Johnson's 1964 "War on Poverty," Canada's Special Planning Secretariat of the Privy Council announced its "war on poverty among the Indians" in 1965. Linking poverty and overcrowding to families with too many children, rather than to house size, the Planning Secretariat sought input from IHS experts. With convoluted logic, the secretariat explained that in a study of the "desirable size of the Indian home under present circumstances" it wondered whether the size of the required prototype home "could be reduced if birth control techniques were actively advocated amongst the Indian population." Read another way, the query's subtext directed that house sizes be reduced in order to compel people to limit family size. In any case, IHS was asked to "express an opinion as to whether birth control techniques would actually affect the size of Indian families in general and hence the size of the house required." Acknowledging the hypothetical nature of the question, since the Criminal Code prohibitions remained, the IHS director sent the inquiry to his senior officers for their opinions on "the medical aspects of the problem and not with theological, legal or other aspects."[72] While most replied that the typical two-room "Indian house" was already so small that it could not be reduced further, many recognized the inquiry as subterfuge to explore the extent of birth control use. The physician-bureaucrats' replies provide a telling commentary on medical attitudes to poverty, reproduction, and the "Indian problem." Their opinions also reflect prevailing notions that the "right" women – the more "advanced" toward assimilation – were already controlling their fertility, while "problem" women required a more coercive approach.

For the most part, bureaucrats, responding promptly to the director's request, supported birth control for their Indigenous patients; likewise, they agreed that the best methods were the ones the professionals could control. J.D. Galbraith at Coqualeetza Indian Hospital in Chilliwack, east of Vancouver, cited with approval the 40 per cent increase in the number of birth control pills prescribed by contracting physicians and supplied from IHS stocks. But, he noted that a certain percentage of women "will not take sufficient care and interest in the regular use of birth control pills" and thus should be fitted with an intrauterine device (IUD). Among these "less co-operative" women he included "unmarried mothers who go on to have sizeable families."[73] Dr M.L. Webb, who had only recently taken over as medical superintendent at North Battleford Indian Hospital in Saskatchewan, agreed that active promotion of birth control techniques would indeed reduce the size of the average family, but that it would take a number of years "depending on how actively one pursued the program." He likewise recommended IUDs for women who would not or could not follow a birth control regime. While he could not see how the already inadequate houses could be made smaller, he argued that "there are many other benefits to be derived from actively pursuing a birth control program, as we well know."[74]

At the Charles Camsell Indian Hospital in Edmonton, medical superintendent Dr G.D. Gray explained that the hospital "advocate[d] for control only after the fifth child has been born, this for medical and socio-economic reasons." Gray did not elaborate on the method of "control," whether sterilization or contraceptives.[75] Dr S. Mallick at the Sioux Lookout Indian Hospital in northern Ontario was more explicit. He explained that the hospital policy was to distribute Enovid birth control pills directly to women with "an excessively large number of pregnancies with no means of support except relief"; for women in poor health "we have carried out sterilization." But Mallick argued that for First Nations women the Pill was less than satisfactory because when a four-month prescription ran out they "are either too late or too lazy to ask for it."[76] Citing favourably the IPPF's use of IUDs in Asia and India, Mallick advocated a large-scale experiment on First Nations women. As a birth control method "more suited" for families with low incomes, the IUD "obviates the necessity and moral objection to sterilization."[77] Hospital-based physicians had considerable authority and opportunity to press their views on women who were deemed to have had "excessive pregnancies." Women who gave birth in IHS Indian hospitals, often far from home, were physically and emotionally vulnerable to such state-sanctioned efforts to control their subsequent reproduction.

Physician-bureaucrats with less direct access to women endorsed the view that Indigenous birthrates indeed required their control; their neo-eugenic solutions focused on the social and economic need to control fertility.[78] Dr T.J. Orford at Regina reckoned that there was no incentive to restrict fertility; indeed, universal social programs and social assistance worked as obstacles: "The man with the large family is in better position to gain by virtue of family allowance and social aid assistance. The female role is, by and large, still that of child bearing."[79] Farther north, at Prince Albert, Saskatchewan, Dr Waldron admitted that some patients "on the more advanced reserves either on the doctor's instructions or at their own request are using birth control tablets and appear to be successful." For many, he continued, education and integration were necessary since they had "no sense of responsibility and the size of the family is of no consequence."[80] The IHS Pacific Region's superintendent, R.D. Thompson, agreed that the "sophisticated and better educated Indians" already used birth control but stated that an effective reduction in the birthrate would only be accomplished by more coercive measures for the isolated and "those of a lower educational standard."[81] At Inuvik, the zone superintendent reported that a good number of both Catholic and non-Catholic patients had prescriptions for the Pill. But, he noted, the abject economic conditions that contributed to continuing high infant-mortality rates convinced many women that it remained necessary to have fourteen children in order for two to survive.[82] Dr R.A. Sprenger in the Yukon Zone endorsed the popular view that medicine's successes, and public health measures in general, raised the standard of living and thus contributed to the current "population explosion." Medicine had a duty to provide education in family planning.[83] IHS bureaucrats' assessments of the "Indian problem" reflected broader middle-class Canadian and international reproductive politics that retained a definite eugenic cast.

The powerful image of "population explosion" as a looming threat to order and stability offered a ready discourse to both explain the problem of poverty in Indigenous communities and provide its solution. In late 1967, despite the legal prohibition, the Northwest Territories Council passed a motion calling on the NWT commissioner to "immediately undertake ... a formal universal and intensive scheme for the dissemination of information about birth control and family planning ... and develop a system through which various birth control devices can be made freely available to anyone wishing them."[84] Framing the problem in the language of population explosion, Lloyd Barber, appointed council member and the dean of commerce at the University of Saskatchewan, urged quick and decisive action to control the birthrate: "Trends imply our population explosion is on a collision course with the ability of the relatively fixed level of renewable resources to support the increasing population."[85] With fewer than thirty thousand people in an area greater than 3.3 million square kilometres, the Northwest Territories were hardly overpopulated.[86] But, as the only Canadian jurisdiction with Indigenous people in the majority, the territorial birthrate was a growing concern for the non-Indigenous council. Characterizing the region's high birth and infant death rates as "Canada's shame," an editorial in the *Edmonton Journal* applauded the NWT Council decision to freely distribute birth control literature and technologies, asking, "Is this India or Latin America?"[87]

DECRIMINALIZATION

In June 1969, the same month that the omnibus Bill C-150 legalizing birth control and abortion became law, Trudeau's Liberal government introduced its "Statement of the Government of Canada on Indian Policy," better known as the White Paper. The timing was not mere coincidence; policy makers in the newly elected government saw themselves as charting a new liberal course for Canadians. Individual choice and individual rights would deliver the social justice and civil rights promised in Trudeau's 1968 "Just Society."[88] The White Paper became a touchstone in national Indigenous political resurgence. Couched in the liberal language of equality and "non-discrimination," the White Paper maintained that First Nations' disadvantaged social, economic, and political position in Canada stemmed not from unfulfilled treaty promises or systemic discrimination but from their different legal status.[89] To create legal equality, the policy proposed to dismantle the Indian Affairs bureaucracy, repeal the Indian Act, and nullify the treaties; it was the logical culmination of the century-long policy of assimilation.[90] Indigenous groups across the country responded with a clear rejection of the badly flawed policy, instead articulating a defence of treaty and Aboriginal rights and demands for greater economic and educational development.[91] The widespread denunciation of the White Paper, supported by the press, led to its withdrawal by early 1971. But its legacy, aside from the impetus for regional groups to organize into a national Indigenous voice, was the deepening distrust of government and a lingering suspicion that termination – or what Harold Cardinal called "cultural genocide" – remained the hidden agenda in policy making.[92] A somewhat chastened bureaucracy learned that to avoid controversy it might consult with community leadership before openly distributing birth control information and technologies. Nevertheless, the amended Criminal Code raised the stakes; reproduction remained a vital state interest and IHS continued its efforts to control Indigenous women's fertility to produce a "normal" family size.

In 1970, the Department of National Health and Welfare established its Family Planning Division, which directed information and public funds to nongovernmental organizations, particularly the FPFC, to promote birth control programs.[93] Provinces had jurisdiction for health services, so the federal government did little more than encourage them to establish birth control services. But, as much as John Munro might have wanted to leave policy to private agencies, in his capacity as federal minister of health he was also the health minister of the Northwest Territories. With its responsibility for health services for Indigenous people, and the NWT Council's now annual motions to develop a "universal and intensive scheme for dissemination of information about birth control and family planning," intended to curb what it deemed unchecked population growth among the Indigenous community, in October 1971 IHS developed its confidential "Family Planning Policy." The policy's "principles and philosophy" for family planning in the "Indian Health Context" began as follows: "balance between population size and available natural resources and productivity is necessary for human happiness, prosperity and peace." The second principle stated that "balance between family size and family income is necessary for raising standards of living and improving health."[94] An individual's right to exercise free choice in the practice of family planning was assured only in principle five (of ten).[95] Not surprisingly, the policy was drafted on the advice of the FPFC and the IPPF, among others.[96] It raises what historian Matthew Connelly calls the critical question of "who would actually do the 'planning' in 'family planning.'"[97]

The IHS policy set out one objective: the reduction of "abnormally high birth rates." It opened by noting that a relationship between the number of "unwanted children" and high infant-mortality rates "probably exists," eliding the question of who considered these children "unwanted." A lowered birthrate would also reduce infant mortality, the incidence of unwanted children, and child abuse and neglect. The policy carefully avoided making a causal link between high birthrates and the consequences, instead implying simply that fewer babies meant fewer problems and an "improvement in family comfort and nutrition." Sexual sterilization was not to be withheld when requested or when deemed medically necessary, as long as both partners understood the "likely result" and signed their consent. The policy memo also noted that advice and explanations might need to be translated into a "native language." Alongside sterilization, the IUD was the only other birth control technology mentioned, and then only to advise that physicians should insert the device (although the following year northern nurses were trained to insert IUDs).[98] The policy promised that family planning would benefit communities but also noted that "its introduction to sensitive native groups could have diverse social, economic, religious and political consequences ... [F]irm backing is therefore necessary from native organizations to avoid commotion." The deputy minister cautioned regional directors to consult with "Native organizations (bands)" before publicly promoting birth control in their communities. However, "low key" efforts should encourage personal demands for medications and contraceptive technologies, which would be met through existing medical and gynecological arrangements and dispensed free of charge.[99]

Even as the Liberals had been preparing their Criminal Code amendments in early 1969, minister of health and welfare John Munro referred to the "genocide question – which arose in a certain form when Harry Cardinal was here." Munro cautioned that the government should avoid mistakes as seen in the United States, where birth control programs were "so obviously pointed at Negro areas." He advised that if the government established openness and credibility in its discussions of birth control aimed at the whole Canadian community, the "message would at least partially get through to subgroups like our Indians."[100] Nevertheless, the 1971 Family Planning Policy, informed by population-control arguments, strove to produce "normal" birthrates. The policy acknowledged that, while some Indigenous communities might welcome their efforts, "others may feel that the strength of the Indian race may be affected."[101] The emergence of revitalized Indigenous political organizations, highly critical of the state, suggested to policy framers that the document should remain "confidential."

Sterilization abuse accusations accompanied the Criminal Code amendments. In early October 1970, MP David Lewis rose in the House of Commons to ask the minister why five Inuit women from the small Arctic community of Holman Island had undergone sterilization, an "unnecessary and inhumane program, in view of the availability of birth control methods."[102] The minister of Indian Affairs, Jean Chrétien, assured the House that the women and their spouses had consented to the procedure after consultation with two physicians.[103] IHS officials explained that requests for sterilization in the North were handled as they were in any province: women consulted their physicians, who would make the determination. The high number was due to a backlog of requests that had built up over a number of years because the only available surgeon was a Roman Catholic who had refused to perform the operation.[104] Lewis, who stated he had no reason to doubt his information, accused the government of forcing women to undergo sterilization. Although IHS bureaucrats insisted that this allegation was unfounded, they immediately refined policy directives to limit access: "Native associations are critical of any methods of birth control being imposed on native people of Canada. They are particularly sensitive about permanent methods of birth control such as tubal ligation and vasectomy." The policy for sterilization reiterated the need for a "definite medical indication" for the procedure, written consent by both partners in the presence of an interpreter and an Indian Affairs welfare officer, and prior bureaucratic approval. Explaining the directive, regional director G.C. Butler stated he did not want to "deny native patients the same rights as non-native" but, in his opinion, Indigenous patients did not understand the implications of sterilization and thus it was "most important that we protect him from his own ignorance in this matter."[105]

CONCLUSION

Class, region, and race shaped women's access to contraceptive information and technologies around the globe in the 1960s and 1970s. The NWT Council's demands for widespread dissemination of birth control in northern Indigenous communities resonated with politicians and "family planning" experts who considered the economic implications of a population explosion too vital an issue to leave to women. White, middle-class physician-bureaucrats developed policy based on the assumption that Indigenous women were not sufficiently motivated to effectively control their own reproduction. Ironically, as soon as birth control was legalized, women's access to it became increasingly constrained. Distribution of birth control information and education, as a part of maternal health care, was limited both by inadequate community healthcare facilities and by concerns that it would provoke an Indigenous nationalist backlash. Coercion under-scored the medical and political discourse of Indigenous women's reproduction. As historian Rebecca Kluchin argues in the American case, contradictory trends of surgical sterilization emerged in the postwar period: white women struggled against pronatalist medical practice to gain access to the technology, while poor women of colour struggled to resist coercive sterilization.[106] In an effort to shield itself from criticism and liability, IHS developed a policy for sterilization of Indigenous women that required the approval of two physicians and the written consent of both partners. Yet, until 1977, IHS policy for the Northwest Territories stated that "all primagravida [first preg-nancy] and grand multiparae (fifth and subsequent infants) [are to be] evacuated to a hospital for delivery as are all complicated preg-nancies or anticipated complications. Provided no complications ensued at the birth of the first infant or if all else is well, second, third or fourth babies are delivered in nursing stations."[107] In unfamiliar hospitals, and often unable to understand the language, Inuit women faced reproductive choices that were routinely compromised by phys-icians, nurses, or private agencies recommending sterilization.[108]

As noted at the outset of this chapter, in early April 1973 CBC Television broadcast an exposé of sterilization abuse of First Nations and Inuit women at the hands of the federal government's IHS. Journalist Charlotte Gobeil interviewed a non-Indigenous woman who had shared a hospital room at Charles Camsell Hospital in Edmonton with a distraught Indigenous woman who was sterilized against her will. Asked why she thought women were being sterilized, "Anna," whose mother had been sterilized, claimed, "I think they're [white people] afraid of the Indian people ... Because a few years ago the Indian people, they were so quiet, but now they are starting to become aware of all their rights ... I work with the Indian Brotherhood of the Northwest Territories, I'm in contact with these Indian people every day, and I think the white people are afraid of the Indian people."[109] Gobeil next interviewed a community chief who suggested that although white people might need population control, in the North "we've got lots of room." A local priest also claimed that the government was intent on a deliberate plan to "cut down on the population as quick as they can" in order to have a free hand to develop the North.

The Canadian North – and, by extension, the Indigenous population – became visible in the 1970s, and federal bureaucrats scrambled to extend their surveillance over this population at the same moment that the state was ostensibly retreating from the domestic spaces of non-Indigenous Canadians. Their actions were buoyed by increasingly intense international debates over the balance of resources and population. In spite of the lack of density in the territories, Canadian officials reasoned that the lack of resources placed that population in circumstances similar to those of the so-called Global South, where more dramatic policies justified aggressive family planning measures to reduce the population bomb that went hand in hand with the war on poverty.

CHAPTER THREE

Indigenous Women in the Provincial South

The 1969 amended Criminal Code brought contraceptive information and technologies out of the shadows and into respectability in the hands of new family planning experts. The next year the federal state created the Family Planning Division to coordinate and promote Canadians' new reproductive autonomy. Never off the agenda was the ideology of the population-control movement that drew a direct line from unchecked reproduction to poverty to global catastrophe. Family planners across the country followed the same logic to identify "high Indian birth rates" (read: Indigenous women) as the existential threat to the nation's future peace and prosperity. At the same time, Red Power militancy brought local issues to a national audience in the global language of decolonization and self-determination. Indigenous women's access to reproductive justice narrowed as population-control anxieties met the gendered nationalisms of Indigenous political activism.

This chapter focuses on how the changing legal landscape created new state and non-state actors who claimed an expertise in planning families, whether their own or others'. The transnational rhetoric of population control that conflated unbridled fertility with poverty and race found a receptive audience in Canada. How this impacted Indigenous women, their families, and their communities is part of a much broader and deeper history of colonialism defined by patriarchal oppression, violence, and trauma. Indeed, the (small) nuclear family model that family planners held up as the ideal was itself the standard that missionaries and residential schools, bureaucrats and the Indian Act, forced on communities in order to undermine Indigenous extended family and clan systems.[1] As settler scholars we are cognizant that our historical methods may be well suited to interpreting settler colonial sources (archival records, published sources, and contemporary press accounts) but are less useful in understanding how communities responded. Our research was not directly informed by communities, though we have incorporated Indigenous voices and scholarly critiques in an effort to demonstrate that Indigenous women have articulated their own responses to these issues, and their perspectives are also contextualized within the contradictory nature of the birth control debates that played out in the 1970s.

Linda Tuhiwai Smith reminds us of the damages that settler research often produces in Indigenous communities.[2] Indigenous scholars employing decolonizing methodologies tell us how women and mothers resist(ed) that oppression by decolonizing womanhood and defining motherhood as empowerment.[3] Reading along, and against, the grain of our sources maps the neo-eugenic assault and its impact on women's choices, but community-based studies would tell a different story of resilience and survival. Population controllers were the latest in a long line of "experts" to undermine Indigenous families in service to a colonialist national agenda.

Canadians learned in 1971 that although its population was only twenty-two million, the nation faced a population crisis. Setting out the state's new priorities, the Family Planning Division's report for Minister Munro alerted Canadians to the looming threat: though birthrates had declined steadily since 1957, Canada's population had doubled between 1933 and 1969, and forecasts suggested it would double again in thirty-five years. Borrowing the language of the global population-control movement, the Family Planning Division predicted that with increasing urbanization, population growth threatened the environment and resources; chaos in overcrowded city slums was not far distant.[4] To forestall that bleak future, Canada needed to heed the lessons of the past. The report explained that since the 1930s, despite the prohibitions in section 150(2)c of the Criminal Code, private birth control clinics and services existed across the country. When the law was tested in Ontario in 1936, nurse Dorothea Palmer, working for eugenicist A.R. Kaufman's Parent's Information Bureau, was acquitted. In his ruling the magistrate cited the inequities in the law that made birth control available to advantaged Canadians but not to the poor and unemployed. By the early 1960s, contraceptives were available in drugstores and doctors freely prescribed oral contraceptives, IUDs, and diaphragms. Citing this history, the Family Planning

Division's report claimed that the law favoured the "highly motivated and more informed members of society." Upper- and middle-class women who could afford the services of a private physician had access to birth control, but for couples "least able to support large families" family planning was an urgent priority.[5] Poor women were seen to lack motivation and clung to superstitious beliefs that birth control was "unnatural," though research suggested they "would like to limit their families to two or three children."[6] The Family Planning Division focused on that goal.

Family Planning's national statistics suggested that Canadians were indeed controlling their fertility: the country's birthrate declined from 26.8 per 1,000 population in 1960 to 17.6 in 1969, and the rate of natural increase (excess of births over deaths) was at its lowest since 1937; the fertility rate was in sharp decline. But, the report warned, the real "population problem" was found in the contrast between national and regional figures, which were influenced by the "native population." The Northwest Territories' natural increase was 31.2 per 1,000 population, or triple the national rate.[7] Within Canada, infant mortality was highest in the two territories. Family Planning identified only one ethnic group; tables labelled "Trend in Indian Birth Rate, 1960–68" and "Trend in Indian Infant Mortality, 1960–69" cited "estimated population" and "estimated births." The statistics, oddly vague, showed falling trends in both categories, but the worrisome figure was a 22 per cent increase in the "Indian" population in the decade.[8] Despite constituting a little more than 1 per cent of Canada's population, Indigenous peoples apparently represented a significant population problem.[9]

Population controller and Edmonton obstetrician Dr Charles Ringrose likened Indigenous communities to "underdeveloped" nations in the Global South where the population was growing at 2 per cent annually while their ability to produce food increased at the rate of just 1 per cent per year: "In our own country, the plight of our native people resembles an underdeveloped nation in that many have insufficient amounts of food of the appropriate quality and their birth rate is very high."[10] Ringrose linked high infant and maternal mortality directly to high birthrates; social problems stemmed from "unwanted children," neglected, abused, and on the path to juvenile delinquency. Much of this would have been greeted with surprise, if not disgust, by his audience – the Voice of Alberta Native Women's Society (VANWS) annual conference. One of Canada's earliest Indigenous political organizations, VANWS worked to temper reserve poverty, overcrowding, inadequate medical care, and the social ills that flowed from residential schooling and the removal of Indigenous children from their families by provincial social workers. "High birthrates" essentially blamed women for the sequela of colonialism or "underdevelopment" in much the same way that the state held women responsible for inadequate housing stock and ill health on reserves. At the conference, Ringrose showed sex education slides and advised that the Pill and IUD were the most effective methods of birth control. The Pill's effectiveness outweighed its side effects, he claimed: "for native women, taking the pill is 50 times safer than having a pregnancy."[11] Speaking in March 1969, on the eve of the Criminal Code amendments, Ringrose foreshadowed the population-control rhetoric that accompanied family planning efforts aimed at Indigenous communities. The title of his talk, "Birth Control – Current Methods of Contraception," promised information and expert advice, but his presentation made clear that expert advice would come wrapped in the accusation that their communities were a population problem.

In the spring of 1972, delegates to the first national conference on family planning, convened by the Department of National Health and Welfare, identified "isolated communities and groups," including Indigenous peoples, as a high priority for family planning programs. The conference recommended that the federal government provide the means for Indigenous people to be trained to provide their communities with family planning information and education in local languages, and that Métis representatives and other associations be invited to future conferences.[12]

Family planning conferences, funded by the federal government and organized by provincial volunteer groups, sprang up across the country in the early 1970s. Conference planners courted local press coverage by featuring speakers who addressed controversial topics like sex education in schools and frank discussions of human sexuality. Like-minded citizens – physicians, nurses, social workers, organized family planning volunteers, women's groups, clergy, and teachers – hammered out resolutions calling for free contraceptives, birth control clinics, and greater access to birth control information and services for those who needed it most. The rhetoric emphasized the need to change attitudes toward, and encourage motivation for, birth control. "Problem groups" included ethnic communities, young people (women), rural residents, the poor, and "native people."[13] The first Alberta Conference on Family Planning, in May 1973, called for free contraceptives for anyone who could not afford them and easier access to tubal ligation, as well as recommending that the government "encourage and actively promote family planning on Reserves."[14]

Many associations that sponsored provincial conferences in the 1970s remained committed to the ideologies of population control, though they had adopted the more benign name of "family planning." The British Columbia Conference, also in May 1973, with 250 participants, was sponsored in part by the BC Family Planning Association (originally the Society for Population Planning, established in 1963). President Mary Bishop and her engineer husband had spent two years in Ceylon (Sri Lanka), where she was exposed to "one of the world's oldest and most densely populated cultures," prompting her activism upon her return to Canada.[15] This was a common path to population-control activism: after a personal brush with "overpopulation," travellers returned "ashen-faced, suitably appalled to tell others of their experience."[16] The BC conference adopted three recommendations aimed at Indigenous people: that "native women Homemakers" be given better financial support and family planning training on the reserves; that community health aides working on reserves be trained in birth control and family planning; and that research should begin on "native medicines traditionally used for contraception purposes ... in order to find out their value, and whether these methods might be more acceptable to native Canadians than methods used for the white population."[17] And, while Bishop herself had three children, the conference urged the Canadian government to adopt a "two child family" population policy.[18]

Indigenous people's reproduction was likewise targeted by the Family Planning Association of Manitoba. The association's constitution outlined its eight objectives: the first, to "encourage good citizenship through responsible family life"; and the next four promising to research the "problems of population growth," to inform the public on the problems of "uncontrolled" population growth, to assist other jurisdictions in their population-control programs, and to take positive action to solve "the world population problem." The lofty goals reflected the intense national and international interest in population control that culminated in the Bucharest Conference and the United Nations declaration of 1974 as World Population Year. But closer to home, the Manitoba planners identified teenagers, "native and métis persons," and "low income persons" as the principal targets of their efforts to control population. Unlike other family planning organizations, however, the Manitoba association included on its board a representative from the Native Women's Association and provided support and training to the Métis Women's Association, which administered its own projects.[19]

Ontario's family planning conference in October 1974, sponsored by Planned Parenthood of Ontario, featured experts from the helping professions and social services, educators, and bureaucrats from three levels of government. Among the 120 delegates were representatives from the Ontario Native Women's Association, Grand Council Treaty 3, Grand Council Treaty 9, the Union of Ontario Indians, and the Association of Iroquois and Allied Indians. They heard speaker Cenovia Addy, federal Family Planning Division consultant, list the target groups whose reproductive bodies needed attention: the poor, "Native" people, young women, and people in rural areas. Whatever else the Indigenous delegates heard at the conference, this alarmed them enough to convene their own workshop arguing that the conference "did not take into consideration the concerns of the Ontario native population in regard to this specific topic."[20] They issued a policy statement with resolutions that made clear that Indigenous organizations would define and address their own needs.

Their resolutions echoed their frustrations with the presumptions of the population controllers and perhaps with experiences with IHS practices. They sketched a plan for communities to build expertise and develop programs within their own organizations around "sex and sexual hygiene education," pointedly eschewing the rhetoric of "family planning." With a share of the funds that were currently directed to Planned Parenthood, Indigenous delegates proposed to design and deliver programs appropriate to their particular communities. Public health and medical staff should be made available only if, and when, Indigenous organizations, associations, or bands requested their services. Priorities and programs would reflect particular Indigenous communities or organizations and should not be understood to apply to all Ontario groups. Finally, the delegates emphasized that neither their presence at the conference nor their resolutions should suggest that all Indigenous communities shared the same views: "We would hope that the Planned Parenthood of Ontario give us the assurance and support to our priorities as defined by our individual boards of directors/councils of our Native organizations, associations or bands."[21] Planned Parenthood's president forwarded the resolutions to the minister of Indian Affairs, since Indigenous peoples were a federal responsibility.[22]

The widespread characterization by social, medical, and government experts of Indigenous communities as problem populations – with, one suspects, "young girls, the poor, and rural residents" often standing in as synonyms – echoed an international rhetoric that equated racialized groups with unrestrained reproduction. Certainly, widely held notions of "unnaturally" high Indigenous birthrates stoked family planners' concerns, yet Indigenous people, comprising only about 1 per cent of Canada's population, were hardly poised to overwhelm the nation. Instead, it seems the threat might have appeared closer to home for urban family planners. The increasing urbanization of Indigenous people, especially after the mid-1960s, added to the spectre of overcrowded city slums breeding social unrest, the very scenario conjured by population controllers' rhetoric about the world's "underdeveloped" Global South.

The colonialist ordering of Canadian space into the 1950s saw most First Nations people settled on reserves and most reserves well removed from urban centres. Segregated settlement patterns began to break down as Indigenous people increasingly moved to cities in search of employment, education, and opportunity.[23] As geographer Evelyn Peters notes, despite relatively small numbers, "city Indians" were perceived by social commentators and all levels of government as "extremely problematic."[24] For example, the Saskatchewan government warned in 1960 that "the day is not far distant when the burgeoning Indian population, now largely confined to reservations, will explode into white communities and present a serious problem indeed."[25] Such concerns centred on the notion that Indigenous people did not belong and could not adapt to urban spaces that were coded modern and non-Indigenous. The "exploding" Indigenous population would have been all too obvious to family planners as they conferred about population problems. Moreover, urban migration in the 1960s and 1970s was accompanied by a resurgent Indigenous activism that brought civil rights and anticolonial liberation movements into a Canadian context.

The politics of reproduction cannot be divorced from the pre– and post–White Paper Indigenous political activism that shifted the political landscape. The National Indian Brotherhood (NIB) emerged in early 1968 as the nascent federation of stronger provincial organizations representing status Indians (those recognized by, and under the authority of, the Indian Act).[26] The Canadian government's White Paper proposals to rescind the Indian Act and terminate the relationship between the federal government and "Indians" thrust the NIB and its leader, Harold Cardinal, onto the national stage. Cardinal's charge that the government was engaged in "cultural genocide" rang true, and the charge would in time be applied to IHS birth control policies.[27] The NIB's surging nationalism in the years after the 1971 withdrawal of the White Paper focused on land claims research, funded with $17 million in government grants by 1976.[28] As well, the more militant Red Power movement also swept the country in the 1970s.

The issues were local, but the Red Power movement's tactics and rhetoric of antiracism and decolonization were transnational.[29] In the summer of 1973, Indigenous youth occupied Department of Indian Affairs offices in Ottawa. A year later, in November 1974, Treaty 7 activists from the Siksika (Blackfoot) reserve east of Calgary, representing the Calgary Urban Treaty Indian Alliance (CUTIA) with involvement of American Indian Movement (AIM), occupied the Indian Affairs office in downtown Calgary.[30] In the summer of 1974, the Ojibway Warriors Society's six-week armed occupation of Anicinabe Park in Kenora, Ontario, had followed the Warriors' occupation of Kenora's Department of Indian Affairs office less than a year earlier.[31] In the fall of 1974, the Native Caravan's cross-country trek from Vancouver to Ottawa culminated in a demonstration and "riot" on Parliament Hill, where police riot squads clashed with mostly unarmed Indigenous men, women, and children.[32] The increasingly militant demonstrations convinced the Trudeau government to establish a consultative Joint Cabinet–National Indian Brotherhood committee in 1975 that linked the NIB executive directly to a special group of cabinet ministers, with the aim of reaching agreement on policy issues.[33]

Urban and militant Indigenous communities also alarmed family planners who saw "population pressure" as the principal social menace facing Canadians. The government physician and population-control advocate at the Fisher River Indian Hospital in Manitoba articulated the dangerous links between political activism, urbanization, and population pressure. He feared women on reserves were being misled and intimidated by "Indian fanatics" like Mohawk activist Kahn-Tineta Horn, who, he claimed, opposed birth control for Indigenous women. Moreover, a focus on Indigenous cultural and linguistic revival and renaissance in schools bred discontent and hatred, all to "satisfy the ego of a few militant Indian leaders." Worse yet, government policies and diminishing employment opportunities on reserves drove young people into cities, creating "red ghettos"; within a generation, Canadian cities would become as unlivable as American cities, with their "negroe [sic] problems." Seemingly all Canadians were imperilled by Indigenous birthrates: "Let us protect our children from a similar fate by doing something now to help the Indian people achieve their goal of equality by giving them a better education and by helping them to space their children and bring the birth rate down."[34] Population controllers adopted the liberal language of "equality" to discipline Indigenous women's fertility in much the same way that the White Paper employed the notion of equality to free "Indians" from the special legal status that presumably kept them from true citizenship.

In the 1970s, Indigenous women's reproduction drew the attention of the neo-eugenic population controllers, while their access to "reproductive justice" – the range of choices that included birth control and abortion but also the freedom to bear and raise their own children – was often mediated by the legacies of residential schools and colonialism. Recalling her mother's experience, Cree/Métis Elder Maria Campbell draws attention to the view of large families as an Indigenous "tradition":

My mom had eight children. When she had her fourth child, the doctor told her she would die if she had more, but she did because she was a Catholic and the church said it was a wife's duty to have babies. My grandmother, who was a traditional healer and midwife, told her she would make her some medicine so she would never get pregnant again. My mom wouldn't take it, and she went on to have three more children. Each one left her weak for months. On her eighth pregnancy my auntie and grandmother pleaded with her to take the medicine. She refused and died, leaving eight children. My grandmother helped many women live to see their grandchildren. She used local plants which were dried and made into tea.[35]

Campbell reminds us that the binary – choice or coercion – is not particularly helpful. References to the "traditionally" large family points to the impact of colonialism and residential schools in not only repressing Indigenous medicine and midwifery that enabled women to control their own fertility but replacing it with Christian morality and ethics that did not.[36]

At the same time, women's political activism advocated for a gendered nationalism and sovereignty that challenged the NIB and its overwhelmingly male leadership. Moreover, women's groups faced chronic funding shortages as Indian Affairs focused its support on the NIB. Indian Affairs provided minimal support (typically one sewing machine each) for the Indian Homemakers' Clubs program that began in 1935. Intended to foster self-improvement and community development, the program also implicitly blamed Indigenous women for reserve poverty and inadequate housing.[37] By the 1970s, Indigenous women's activism sought wider political organizations that focused on social justice, equality, and education. Yet, Indian Affairs refused to financially support women's organizations that "operate at the provincial or national level ... or those whose function is primarily political."[38] In 1968, Mrs Rose Charlie, of Sts'Ailes (Chehalis, BC), united the provincial homemakers' clubs into the BC Indian Homemakers' Association (BCIHA), with a heterogeneous membership representing urban and reserve women, independent of Indian Affairs.[39] As part of its mandate, the BCIHA distributed information on counselling, guidance, and general assistance to women regarding the health and welfare needs of women and children, including information kits on reproductive health and birth control access.[40] The official organ of the BCIHA, the *Indian Voice* newspaper (established in 1969), advocated for change at the grassroots level and centred women within the discourse of Indigenous nationalism. The *Voice* depicted male leaders as indifferent to local issues, while women were portrayed as rooted in their Indigenous identity as female citizens of their Nations.[41] By the 1970s, the department of the Secretary of State provided some funding for Indigenous women's groups, but its funding model further hobbled Indigenous women activists by limiting support to groups that represented all women regardless of legal Indian status. Those groups that mounted the most sustained challenge to the NIB leadership – such as Indian Rights for Indian Women (IRIW), which focused solely on the repeal of the Indian Act's sex discrimination clause – could find little support from status Indian women and therefore were left without any funding.

Under section 12(I)(b) of the Indian Act, a status woman who married a non-Indian man lost her status, as did her children, while an Indian man who married a non-Indian woman retained his status, and his wife and her children became "Indian." In *Indian Women and the Law in Canada: Citizens Minus*, Kathleen Jamieson describes the consequences for Indigenous women:

> The woman, on marriage, must leave her parents' home and her reserve. She may not own property on the reserve and must dispose of any property she does hold. She may be prevented from inheriting property left to her by her parents. She cannot take any further part in band business. Her children are not recognized as Indian and are therefore denied access to cultural and social amenities of the Indian community. And most punitive of all, she may be prevented from returning to live with her family on the reserve, even if she is in dire need, very ill, a widow, divorced or separated. Finally, her body may not be buried on the reserve with those of her forebears.[42]

In 1970, when Jeannette Vivian Corbiere, a Nishnawbe woman from the Wikwemikong Reserve on Manitoulin Island in Ontario, married David Lavell, a non-Indigenous man, she lost her status. She took her challenge as far as the Supreme Court of Canada, arguing that the Indian Act discriminated on the basis of sex and race.[43] The political implication of the court challenge was that if the Indian Act were deemed racist and struck down by the court, it would accomplish judicially what the White Paper could not accomplish politically. In what scholar Sally Weaver sarcastically calls a "remarkable demonstration of unity," the NIB and each of its provincial organizations intervened in the Supreme Court case *against* Lavell.[44] Ultimately, the Supreme Court ruled in 1973 against Lavell, leaving the Indian Act's discriminatory clause intact for another twelve years. It also cast the Indigenous women's equal rights movement as "anti-Indian" and a direct challenge to the NIB's nationalist aspirations.[45] Cree activists Nellie Carlson and Kathleen Steinhauer recall that the long fight for equality divided families and communities; privately, Harold Cardinal admitted they were right, but he would not support them publicly, while "some other men would make fun of what they called 'squaw lib.'"[46] Activist Colleen Glenn suggested that Cardinal's leadership, and his opposition to changing the Indian Act, influenced the federal government more than women could: "I remember being in a meeting ... with cabinet ministers when [Indian Act] section 12(1)(b) was brought up. And [then cabinet minister] Marc Lalonde said, 'The men wanted it that way.'"[47]

Women faced the colonizing state as well as the patriarchy of their respective national organizations: "the brotherhoods" and their nationalist agendas. As Métis scholar Emma LaRocque notes, colonialism and nationalism are gendered, such that in nationalist movements "women are celebrated abstractly as carriers of culture and guardians of tradition" while their fundamental rights are often denied. In moments of nationalism, women are most vulnerable to fundamentalisms and disempowerment.[48] Cree-Métis scholar Kim Anderson acknowledges that given colonialism's attacks on Indigenous bodies and families through sterilizations, residential schools, and child welfare interventions, pronatalism was a not unreasonable response. But she also links pronatalism with liberation movement ideologies that typically "confine women to motherhood roles within the patriarchal family."[49] As we have seen, population-control ideologies heavily influenced the federal government's 1971 policy "Family Planning in the Indian Health Context." But in the face of increasing nationalistic demands by (male) Indigenous political activists, senior bureaucrats warned against promoting birth control in communities without the approval of political organizations, "to avoid commotion."[50]

Indigenous women's "choice" of access to birth control information and technologies was further mediated at the local level by the personal, political, and religious convictions of band politicians, physicians, and bureaucrats. When Indigenous communities in British Columbia raised concerns about inadequate and overcrowded housing, the regional bureaucrat identified a lack of family planning, not too few houses, as the principle problem: "We believe that this overcrowding is one of the most serious hazards to community health and this is of course combined with the economic disadvantages of caring for large families. Our opinion is that Family Planning would very greatly assist in improving the health status of many communities both Indian and white."[51] But his superior judged that family planning information was too sensitive to discuss openly; instead, it might be raised with band councils, to inform them that IHS staff would provide information "at their request."[52] A senior bureaucrat in British Columbia (who presumed to know what women wanted) complained about the policy:

Indian women are interested in family planning, and the Pill and IUD is [sic] quite acceptable to them. The present problem is that while we are allowed to give information on a one to one basis on request, we are not permitted to give talks or hold seminars. The result is that the women who have most need of the information are the ones who never hear about it and who do not request information. Let's face the fact that it is politics (both Government and Indian Associations) and not acceptability that is hindering progress in this matter.[53]

Of course, not all communities heeded the supposed political dictates of national leadership. In 1974, the Native Women's Association of Manitoba published a popular pamphlet directed at Indigenous couples, *Family Planning and Birth Control Methods*. Couched in terms of individual family choice, the pamphlet outlined in clear language the strengths and weaknesses of available contraceptive devices and procedures.[54]

The contradictions in policy, between population-control rhetoric that blamed women for "abnormal birth rates" and the paternalism that ensured politicians and bureaucrats controlled access to information, left women particularly vulnerable. Ultimately, women had to navigate those contradictions in the privacy of the examination room and on terms and conditions not of their own making. Physicians' insights into the examination-room encounter dominate in the archival record, where their paternalism is unquestioned and uneven power relations are taken as normal and natural. Nevertheless, these encounters offer a glimpse into the everyday politics of reproduction.

A husband and wife team arrived as medical officers at the Fisher River Indian Hospital in Manitoba in 1965. They stayed for five years and left a self-serving memoir (in the husband's voice) highly critical of government mismanagement of the "Indian problem." The single greatest problem on all reserves, the doctor proclaimed, was the high birthrate: "It is pure nonsense to tell me that the Indian woman wanted more children and thus we should help them to have large families. Nothing could be further from the truth. Once the communication barrier is broken, we found the great majority of Indian women did not want a baby every year. They have similar aspirations and desires as any non-Indian."[55] The hospital kept a special card file to document patients' regular pap smears and for "family planning purposes." According to the memoir, local women did not initially request birth control pills until they understood the new physicians' stance on family planning, after which pills were offered from the hospital's large stock to each mother after she had given birth at the hospital. When the local United Church minister invited the doctor to give a talk on family planning in 1965, the doctor recalled, his superiors warned him to decline because advocating the use of birth control remained against the law. He called the law inhumane and the work of "bigots and hypocrites."

While departmental policy limited discussions of family planning to individual counselling behind closed doors, it permitted physicians to request permission to perform tubal ligations on women "who had too many children" and those with serious obstetrical complications. The Fisher River doctor's first "test case" was a thirty-six-year-old woman with numerous pregnancies and a history of serious postpartum bleeding. The sterilization committee at a Winnipeg hospital approved the surgery and the patient returned home without complications after a few days. With obvious pride, the physician recalled that every year he sent four or five women to Winnipeg for sterilization; more than fifty women were on the Pill and another thirty fitted with IUDs. He claimed to have cut the birthrate by 35 per cent by 1968. However, he regretted that teen pregnancy continued, with about ten girls per year forced to leave school to have "unwanted" babies and become (he assumed) welfare recipients. He offered to provide sex education in the school, but officials would only do so upon parents' request; the parents were "not sophisticated enough" to allow it.

In one instance, however, the physician recalled that he had "obtained consent" from a woman (and her husband) for tubal ligation after her current pregnancy. Upon return from her confinement in Winnipeg the woman stopped at the Indian hospital to register her shock at the attempt to perform surgery. "They wanted to cut me open, so I came home," she said. Disgusted with medical care, she refused to spend another minute in the Indian hospital and stepped out into the November night with her five-day-old infant to walk to her home reserve miles away. Her "consent" to the surgery had clearly not been informed, and she'd had the wherewithal to refuse the surgery. Indeed, departmental consent forms failed to describe either the procedure or the process and were designed to absolve surgeons of legal liability:

I do hereby request and consent to the performance of an operation upon myself for the purpose of preventing me from becoming pregnant in the future. I agree and bind myself and my heirs and anyone representing me not to bring or cause to be brought any action for damages or otherwise against any physician, surgeon or any other party engaged or concerned in the performance of such an operation or for any resulting consequences or effects arising out of the said operation.[56]

One can imagine the difficulty in translating the form's barely comprehensible legalese into Indigenous languages, if indeed any attempts were made.

In the wake of the very public charges that Indigenous women were sterilized without their knowledge or consent, bureaucrats clarified policies at Indian hospitals. Hospitals were directed to have interpreters available and to translate consent forms into Indigenous languages, though problems continued with both the limited information used in the consent forms and the quality of translations. On the other hand, women's access to birth control and abortion became more constrained as bureaucrats feared public controversy and an Indigenous nationalist backlash. While the unified women's movement in Canada had developed in opposition to restricted access to abortion under the 1969 Criminal Code, Indigenous women saw their access even more limited under the new law.[57] The IHS informed the Badgley Committee on the Operation of the Abortion Law that "there is no particular problem with regard to Indians and Eskimos and abortions. In the past, there have been occasional claims by some national groups (particularly Indians) that deliberate genocide is being carried out by the performance of abortions on Indians and Eskimos. These claims have been looked into in great detail and do not have any validity."[58] Nevertheless, few Indian hospitals had the necessary hospital accreditation to establish the requirements that would prompt a therapeutic abortion committee to approve the procedure, and even fewer provided abortions.[59]

At Edmonton's Charles Camsell Hospital, Indigenous women seeking abortions needed not only a request from their attending physician but also a letter of recommendation by an impartial consultant in spite of the concurrence of the TAC. The hospital took "extra-ordinary precautions with this particular group of patients as compared to the routine caucasian [sic] office patient."[60] No abortions were performed at Moose Factory Hospital in northern Ontario, where tubal ligation required the written consent of two consultants as well as the consent of the patient's husband.[61] Especially in northern and rural regions, reproductive health care was only available in government hospitals, where administrators limited women's access to procedures to avoid controversy. The federal deputy minister of health was informed that public discussions of family planning were ineffective and "have in the past, and can still be interpreted as having overtones of genocide."[62] For many Indigenous women, access to basic birth control information remained limited to the occasional visit by a public health nurse or after the birth of her baby.

Reproductive politics shifted in the 1970s as liberalizing legislation promised greater autonomy for Canadian adults. Yet, Indigenous women's reproduction came under greater scrutiny when Canadian experts fused the international movement for population control with poverty and racialized women. Accompanied by increasing urbanization, activists' protests against racism and discrimination seemed to confirm the worst fears of population controllers: high birthrates leading to social unrest. In what Johanna Schoen calls the "Jekyll-and-Hyde nature" of state involvement in reproductive policies, some Indigenous women lost autonomy over their reproduction when, hospitalized for childbirth, they were pressured into sterilization by physicians who judged they had too many children; some gained autonomy when access to birth control coincided with physicians' willingness to dispense technologies and devices.[63] Nevertheless, some women struggled to define a gendered notion of Indigenous citizenship that clashed with the aspirations of nationalist politicians, particularly over the Indian Act. At some times and in some places, talk of genocidal policies drowned out open access to birth control information while Indigenous self-determination recalibrated the politics of reproduction.

CHAPTER FOUR

Sex and Responsibility in the Community

Canada's formal eugenics programs included Alberta's Sexual Sterilization Act, in place from 1928 to 1972 and responsible for the sterilization of nearly three thousand people, fifty-five of whom were sterilized during the final year of the program.[1] British Columbia passed a similar law in 1933 that was repealed forty years later, in 1973; however, compared with Alberta, the BC program never enjoyed full support, meaning that the development of a comprehensive institutional network and allotment of administrative resources to the program were limited. The scant archival record that remains suggests that approximately two hundred women were sterilized in British Columbia; we found no men listed in the official records. The Law Reform Commission of Canada (LRCC) reported in 1979 that these programs had been justified in part in an effort to relieve the economic burden of long-term care and social services. But that commission also outlined three distinct advantages to nonconsensual sterilization: "removal of the threat of parenthood with which the mentally handicapped may be unable or unprepared to cope; inability of the mentally handicapped to bear the financial burden that accompanies rearing children; and for reasons of personal hygiene."[2]

Mental hygiene movements emerged in the early twentieth century as a progressive response to mental illness and psychiatric disorders. The eugenics movement subscribed to preventive measures, to avoid or at least minimize the risk of becoming mentally ill. By the 1920s several jurisdictions in North America and Europe had merged the science of eugenics into mental hygiene movements, meaning that the key targets for eugenic sterilization were people with mental, intellectual, or physical disabilities. Indeed, when Nazi Germany passed its first sterilization policy in 1933, it was titled the Law for the Prevention of Offspring with Hereditary Diseases. The focus on preventing these conditions relied on hereditary science that linked such diseases or defects with inheritable conditions. It also gave significant power and authority to the psychiatry profession to define categories of disease and their likelihood of transmission through reproduction. Given these conditions, during the first half of the twentieth century, eugenics and mental hygiene dominated discussions of birth control, framing it as a progressive means of reducing the rate of mental illness and disability.

During World War II, eugenics policies assumed a new scale, becoming connected to the Holocaust and coercive measures that targeted people beyond clinical categories. In the postwar reconstruction effort, the international community agreed that this approach to prevention and mental hygiene was too susceptible to abuse. Despite concerns raised at the Nuremburg Trials investigating the conditions for human experimentation, many non-German jurisdictions remained confident that their approaches were different, still guided by sound scientific principles, and therefore continued practising eugenic sterilization with a focus on preventing disability. The rhetoric, however, slowly gave way to concerns about responsibility and parenthood, or dependency on the state or welfare institutions, over more explicit worries about passing on hereditary material through reproduction. By the 1960s and 1970s the logic more readily concentrated on social and environmental conditions but retained a focus on birth control and sterilization as a genuine tool for preventing the spread of these conditions.

These claims about irresponsible parenthood echoed eugenic ideas but shifted the onus from hereditary causes to social and economic ones. The legal justifications continued to rely on the concept of eugenics, or, as some scholars have more recently suggested, a form of "newgenics" – that is, the continuation of eugenic logic in the 1970s with new vocabulary or updated terminology suggestive of a break with the form of eugenics more commonly associated with Nazi fascism. Some activists suggest that by using the term "newgenics" we acknowledge the connections to the eugenic past and recognize that postwar strategies to control fertility or remove children from parents with intellectual or psychiatric diagnoses is indeed a continuation of eugenic practices.[3] Historically, eugenics reformers argued that despite the discredited science of eugenics, the notion that people with mental disorders were unfit parents remained paramount and helped to justify continued surveillance of their sexual activities in an effort to prevent future generations of people with mental disorders, low intelligence scores, mental deficiencies, or a litany of disorders and disabilities that might fall under the umbrella of undesirable behaviours.

Although only two Canadian provinces had formal laws regarding nonconsensual sterilization, the practice of sterilizing people against their will was much more widespread. Psychiatric and training school facilities in eastern Canada had long engaged in the segregation of women of childbearing age in the mental health system in an effort to control pregnancy.[4] Ontario had relied on similar approaches but in 1964 began widely using Depo-Provera injections on an experimental basis to stop menstruation for up to fourteen weeks in fertile women confined to institutions.[5] The rationale behind these practices remained consistent with claims outlined by the LRCC, reinforcing the idea that the state ought to play a role in preventing pregnancy among this population of people considered too ill or too incapacitated to make decisions for their own benefit.

In this chapter we build on some of the historical literature that explores how ideas of eugenics transformed in the second half of the twentieth century and commingled with ideas of reproductive health.[6] The historiographical focus on eugenics in Canada has emphasized the activities in British Columbia and Alberta, provinces that maintained eugenics programs into the 1970s.[7] This literature is generally separate from the historiography on deinstitutionalization, disability, and the changing contours of Canada's mental health system in the 1970s, but we bring both together here to highlight how conceptions of mental health continued to condition reproductive choices. In this chapter we interpret how eugenic ideas and the politics of choice collided in the 1970s, particularly for individual women considered incapable of making rational choices. We focus on the public debates that unfolded in Ontario and concentrated on discussions about disability, sexuality, and responsibility during the age of community care. Newspaper reports and government correspondence suggest that releasing people from custodial care to community care also triggered concerns about whether people with disabilities living in autonomous or semi-autonomous homes might be either subject to sexual abuse or incapable of responsible parenting. Parents urged the Ontario Health Insurance Program (OHIP) to cover the cost of sterilizing adult children with disabilities, and lawyers interpreted the obligations of the medical profession with respect to this issue. Before the recognition of HIV/AIDS in the early 1980s, and prior to the introduction of the Canadian Charter of Rights and Freedoms, rights-based discussions concerning disability focused on preventing people from engaging in sexual behaviour, which was justified as a form of protection.

REPEALING EUGENICS LAWS

By the 1970s, the context of debates over reproductive rights had changed significantly. British Columbia and Alberta had established sexual sterilization programs at a time when all contraception and abortion was illegal, before World War II, meaning that advocates for both coercive and voluntary forms of birth control and fertility restriction made broad use of the concept of eugenics. The federal government's Criminal Code amendments in 1969 relaxed laws on contraception, including allowances for sterilization for such purposes, and abortion, thus offering some supporters of eugenics the opportunity to claim victory, both morally and politically, for birth control's decriminalization. Eugenics, however, had become tarnished by its association with the Holocaust and with draconian images of coercive sterilizations, primarily those occurring in the thousands in psychiatric and penal institutions around the world.[8] But while the word "eugenics" came to connote an image of paternalistic control over marginalized bodies, second-wave feminists embraced the same technologies and rebranded them as a means of liberation from those same patronizing forces.

According to the Edmonton-based Institute of Law Research and Reform, "The repeal in 1972 of the Sexual Sterilization Act ... ended a dark chapter in the history of the mentally disabled in Alberta. Drafted to protect the gene pool with no consideration of individual rights, this Act had allowed sterilization of mentally disabled persons without their consent. This discredited legislation has contributed greatly to the political sensitivity of this issue; no one wants a return to what amounted to forced sterilization."[9] Legal inquiries in the 1970s emphasized that science and the law had moved beyond the crude approximations of human inheritance and intelligence that had once guided the architects of eugenics programs. The legal reports implied that future clinical interventions, including sterilizations, would be better informed by scientific evidence and sound public policy that prioritized the rights of individuals more directly over the concerns of the state.

Alberta was in some ways on the hot seat in these debates, having defended its eugenics program as recently as 1968, claiming that it had saved the province money and been built on sound scientific evidence.[10] Leading geneticists disputed the latter claim, but the Social Credit government remained committed to the program until its defeat in 1971 by the Conservatives, who quickly moved to dismantle it. In 1978, however, that same government introduced the Dependents Adult Act, a new law that allowed parents and guardians of people declared mentally incompetent to recommend sterilization on their behalf. This option of electing certain individuals for nontherapeutic sterilization surgery was in keeping with mainstream society's menu of contraceptive choices, but the creation of a third-party decision-making structure complicated the situation.

The revised law allowed sterilizations to continue on a population of individuals in psychiatric facilities and those considered mentally incompetent, with the newly added layer of consent by proxy or consent from parents or guardians, echoing the stipulation in certain jurisdictions requiring permission from a husband or the recommendation of a therapeutic abortion committee. Once again, Alberta made some bold legal strides by codifying these practices in law, but other jurisdictions embraced similar practices without passing specific policies. For example, on 24 April 1973 an employee of the Metropolitan Toronto Association for the Mentally Retarded proposed that anyone seeking financial support for sheltered or subsidized housing on account of mental disability should be sterilized as a condition of their acceptance into that funding program. Although the Ontario director of such facilities opposed the proposal, those objections were overruled, and the director was later forced to resign for not supporting the organization.[11] That same year female trainees, or patients, of the Ontario Hospital [Training] School at Cedar Springs were denied tubal ligations at the local general hospital. The patients were all over the age of eighteen but deemed incapable of giving informed consent. In this instance, the hospital struck a committee on behalf of the "retarded patient," as defined in the report, to adjudicate these requests on a case-by-case basis.[12] This example is thus another variation of the third-party consent requirement that appears following the federal government's 1969 Criminal Code amendments.

In Ontario, psychiatrists and policy makers also debated the relative merits of downsizing long-stay custodial facilities, a practice that was widespread across North America, but in doing so confronted the reality that sterilization surgeries had been occurring within psychiatric and custodial facilities as part of a treatment plan. Sterilization procedures in Ontario were carried out predominantly on women; the argument went that some women were disabled to such an extent that they were incapable of taking care of their own menstruation. As a result, personal or menstrual hygiene became an additional challenge for staff in charge of several patients or residents – and to improve the efficiency of the institution, teenage women living in these facilities were sterilized to prevent them from menstruating.

Beginning in the mid-1960s these institutional facilities began closing or downsizing and institutionalized people were expected to live independently, semi-independently, or with considerable outpatient care in the community. Sterilizing them in the community, however, presented new challenges. Patients and (ex-)patient activists lobbied for more autonomy and were recognized, at least in part, for stimulating the move out of institutions in the first place. Policy makers and healthcare professionals were divided on how best to balance personal autonomy with concerns for hygiene as well as reproduction and sexual abuse in the community. Two key Ontario players emerged in these debates: Dennis Timbrell, Ontario's health minister; and Donald Zarfas, a psychiatrist practising in Hamilton. Timbrell drew a firm line in the sand by stating that no person in this category of disability should be sterilized. His argument was exactly opposite that of early eugenics reformer Emily Murphy, who had stated that "no insane person should be entitled to progeny."[13] Zarfas, another vocal and public advocate for deinstitutionalized people, sharply disagreed with Timbrell; instead, he argued that any decisions on sterilization must consider, on a case-by-case basis, the sexual and family desires of these former patients as well as input from those who care for them on a day-to-day basis, their physician, and even a neutral community observer. These public comments by Zarfas and Timbrell on the issue of sterilization for people with mental, intellectual, and physical disabilities helped to complicate the public understanding of the issue. The discussions also articulated some of the legal framework for determining competency and assigning responsibility for the alleged problem of sexuality and reproduction for disabled people living in the community.

By the end of the 1970s, Timbrell had recommended abolishing all sterilizations of minors and individuals with mental disabilities, both categories of people he insinuated were incapable of providing free and informed consent. The LRCC softened this proposal, declaring that mentally incompetent individuals should not be sterilized "against their will."[14] A March 1978 article in the *Globe and Mail* argued that sterilizations of children were necessarily against their will and should unilaterally be illegal.[15] Although Timbrell admitted that the province required more information before formulating policy on the matter, the NDP social services critic, Ross McClellan, claimed that "the sterilizations represent a monumental violation of the human rights of retarded persons."[16] Meanwhile, John Sweeney of the government's social development committee argued that "sterilizations indicate a buildup of retarded people being abused in one sense or another."[17] However, how those abuses were defined, and how consent and choice were assigned, continued to complicate the matter.

In Quebec, legislators debated the same issues. Dr David Roy of Montreal's Centre for Bioethics made the case that "we need to protect the rights and respect the needs and capabilities of the mentally handicapped, in considering the sterilization of these individuals."[18] Roy was speaking to an assembly of physicians, parents, theologians, and policy makers at a two-day conference devoted to the topic, with the express purpose of later informing the provincial government on the matter. Quebec had carried out between 250 and 300 sterilizations in 1978, about half the number that had occurred in Ontario in the same period. Ultimately, the Montreal meeting explored a multilayered decision-making apparatus: "a decision-making process should take all factors, including the support the person needs to live and the right to sexual and emotional expression into account."[19] Extending the context of decision-making, as well as the consequences of both sterilization and reproduction, the conversation in Quebec moved beyond the idea of competency to also consider the nature of support available.

Each province struggled in its own way to draw a clear legal line that distinguished competency from incompetency as it pertained to consent for surgeries, combining procedures that resulted in sterilization, experimentation, transplantation, and psychosurgery. Rather than defer decision-making to parents or guardians, the LRCC recommended the transfer of authority to a multidisciplinary board, "composed of such people as physicians, lawyers, social workers, psychiatrists, and representatives of the public."[20] The commission ultimately looked to clinical professionals to make "ethical" choices on behalf of institutionalized or recently deinstitutionalized patients of childbearing age.

The legal arm of the medical profession, the Canadian Medical Protective Agency (CMPA), quickly weighed into the debates, particularly out of concern for the impact of these decisions on physicians. One CMPA official explained that "there are those who believe sterilization of a mentally retarded person is an infringement on civil liberties of the person and that consent for it cannot be properly given by anyone." He continued by offering legal advice: "although we do not wholly agree with this point of view it must be acknowledged nevertheless that there may be groups or individuals who object strenuously to the principle of sterilization because of mental incapacity." Ultimately, the CMPA concluded that "the Association has concurred with decisions for sterilization of mentally retarded minors" in cases where the parents recommended the operation.[21]

Adding parents into an otherwise patient-physician relationship triangulated the decision-making process. Yet this triad of players was familiar to people experiencing institutional life where patients or residents of long-stay facilities rarely had autonomy over their own decisions, even under guidance from physicians. Now the decisions lay primarily with parents, who were increasingly responsible for the daily care and/or expense of daily care for their impaired child. As Michel Desjardins explains, double standards are considerable when it comes to assessing sexuality in people labelled intellectually disabled; their sexuality becomes subject to "a series of extraordinary rules, controls, and prohibitions," including sterilizations, framed as a progressive intervention that permits nonprocreative sex.[22]

Zarfas, a former superintendent of the Ontario Hospital School for Children and expert on pediatric "mental retardation," argued that parents were among the most likely to recommend sterilization and consequently should not be given this legal position. Instead, he argued that children and teens needed advocates and third-party decision-makers to make ethical decisions about their sexual and reproductive lives. Zarfas was a clear advocate for sterilization, but he stood apart from many of his contemporaries who suggested that individuals with disabilities and low intelligence should be sterilized because of the likelihood of irresponsible parenthood. He argued instead that wide variation existed in the capacity to parent among this population and that neither front-line healthcare staff nor parents were in the best position to judge. Zarfas suggested that such a decision "should be [made by] someone who can stand back, 'stand in the shoes of' and protect the rights of the retarded person." He recommended the role of psychologist Wolf Wolfensberger's "citizen advocate": "a *citizen* advocate – not a lawyer advocate – someone who could represent the retarded person as an individual."[23] Importantly, Zarfas felt that family members should be consulted but not left to make these decisions, as they often "panic" about their own responsibilities associated with an unwanted pregnancy. In other words, he pushed back against the CMPA's recommendation that parents should shoulder responsibility for decisions about sterilization because he felt that parents of disabled children feared pregnancy more than anyone. But, by emphasizing this feature, Zarfas also contributed to a shift in the discourse that refocused on women as the main subjects for consideration by linking the notion of responsibility to parenting and pregnancy. This shift in the 1970s to focusing on women in the debates also changed the tenor of the conversation from the earlier days of discussing eugenic sterilization. Although numbers in provincial cases had varied, the gender distribution in the Alberta eugenics program favoured women only slightly over men, but by the 1970s sterilizations in custodial institutions across Canada were performed predominantly on women.

In the early 1970s, as noted, Wolfensberger introduced the concept of a citizen advocate. He aggressively promoted a theory of normalization, especially concerning individuals with intellectual disabilities who were in the 1970s being moved into community settings with greater regularity. A fierce champion of individual rights and assimilation into the community, Wolfensberger's ideas resonated in Ontario with fellow advocates like Zarfas who both supported care in the community but also recognized a need for new policies or practices for managing sexuality in this context.[24]

Zarfas's position reveals some of the edges of the debate in this period, as it straddled issues of personal autonomy, personal (including menstrual) hygiene, and parental authority. He vehemently advocated for the humanizing of people who had long been institutionalized, which remained in line with the principle of deinstitutionalization that emphasized the need for people to be cared for in the community. That move, however, reflected long-standing fears about people with disabilities or psychiatric illnesses returning to the community and the need to protect them from sexual predation. In addition, the underlying logic implied that people could not or would not engage in *protected* sex, may be subjected to sexual predation and abuse, and furthermore would be incapable of raising children. Children born to a parent or parents who were considered to have compromised mental functioning were perceived to be incapable of reaching full independence through a combination of genetic and environmental influences. That is, whether they inherited so-called biological defects or whether the nurturing from a disabled parent compromised their upbringing, children born into these circumstances were considered less likely than other children to develop into independent adults. Among these influences, but rarely if ever mentioned explicitly, remained a firm conviction among policy makers and reformers that those born into a life of poverty were unlikely to overcome this economic condition. Although the notion of responsible parenting might have been expanded to include other elements, the discussions centred on links between personal responsibility and dependence on welfare, or dependence on the state. Given that by the 1970s it was already clear that ex-psychiatric patients disproportionately lived below the poverty line, this connection took on additional meaning: poverty could be pathologized.

EUGENICS AND INSTITUTIONS

While parents with dependent children argued that they needed tailored support to care for their adolescent children at home, custodial psychiatric and long-term care institutions continued to insist that sexuality, fertility, and menstrual hygiene presented challenges for working conditions. One Kingston-based physician claimed that "fertility is a problem which must be faced at institutions for the mentally retarded ... [W]e have to be concerned about sexuality and fertility in these government-operated residences."[25] As contraceptive pills came under public scrutiny in the early 1970s for their dangerous side effects, including headaches, blood clots, and even strokes, the idea of surgical solutions to fertility for people living in institutions became more palatable.

In December 1978, headlines in the *Globe and Mail* informed readers that people with psychiatric or intellectual disabilities were continuing to be sterilized and, moreover, that local Ontario support staff were encouraging these operations. News of sexual sterilizations occurring in psychiatric and custodial institutions were reminiscent of eugenics and a history of coercive sterilizations, but while the surgical procedures remained consistent, the rationale had changed. Rena Paul, a social worker and former director of family services for the Metropolitan Toronto Association for the Mentally Retarded, said, "Sterilization is the only method of birth control for mentally retarded people ... I'm worried that a suspension of sterilization will again lead to the segregation of mentally retarded men and women. These people should have the freedom to [have] sexual contact and to enjoy each other's company."[26] Paul had already published a report in a legal journal, coauthored with University of Toronto law professor Bernard Green, where they had articulated a deeper set of concerns for the need to offer sterilization operations to people with cognitive impairments now living in the community. Paul and Green estimated that in Ontario, over two hundred thousand people had been released from custodial facilities under the guiding premise of "normalization." The principles of normalization suggested that such people should be able to lead "normal" lives and be supported in doing so. Part of that process, according to Paul, Green, and many others, was to allow former patients to engage in sexual relations, or marriage, and to express their sexuality freely and without judgment. However, Paul and Green also concluded that reproduction within this population created a very high risk of transmission of disability. Referring to a 1965 study from the Minnesota Human Genetics League, they suggested that "1 to 2 per cent of the population composed of fertile retardates, produced 36.1 per cent of the retardates of the next generation ... The fact that about five-sixths of the retarded have a retarded parent or a retarded aunt or uncle is of great significance because it demonstrates the large extent to which transmission is involved in the etiology of mental retardation."[27]

The argument for sexual freedom added a significant new dimension to the controversy that had long plagued discussions of sexuality and reproduction among institutionalized people. The divergent perspectives on sexual rights further complicated the idea that the law and, by extension, medicine had a responsibility to protect these so-called vulnerable citizens. The concerns raised in the *Globe and Mail*, therefore, tapped into a wider set of debates across the country as to how to balance the rights of disabled individuals with the internal and administrative function of institutions alongside fears of disease and disability transmission in the community.[28]

By the end of the 1970s, the issue of sterilization surgery for adolescent children with severe mental and physical disabilities was attracting more publicity and becoming the focus of a review by the LRCC, which aimed at providing legal guidance on the ethics of sterilization. Among the variety of proposals it received from across Canada was Minister Timbrell's aforementioned recommendation to abolish all sterilizations on people with diagnosed psychiatric or intellectual disorders. Timbrell's proposal followed the release of a report by Zarfas, who was by then a special consultant on mental retardation with the Ontario Ministry of Community and Social Services. Zarfas's report indicated that, in the absence of a clear policy on the matter, 608 individuals deemed mentally incompetent had been sterilized in 1976 without their consent, although the hospitals concerned had obtained consent from those patients' next of kin. Only 50 of those sterilized were men or boys, reinforcing a gender imbalance in these cases.[29] The *Medical Tribune* repeated this information, publishing a short article that drew attention to the contradiction between the law and practice, quoting an Ontario government lawyer who stated that "minors, and people institutionalized as mentally infirm, were being sterilized ... in substantial numbers" illegally.[30] Mr Perry, the lawyer interviewed for this case, suggested that although Ontario was engaged in these kinds of practices and may have sterilized approximately 8,000 people in 1978, Alberta and British Columbia had (and here he speculated, incorrectly) also sterilized approximately 8,000 people through their eugenics laws; further, he believed 6,500 of those people were "Native Indians."[31] Albertan reports later disputed this claim, but the argument here seems to suggest that Ontario's practices had been no more severe than those in the two provinces with eugenic sterilization laws in place.

In a letter to parents of children who attended the New Dawn School, designed for children with intellectual and physical disabilities, the principal relayed the Ontario government's decision to place a "moratorium on sterilization of children under 16."[32] The letter acknowledges a legacy of past abuses and makes a clear statement about the need to let parents decide such matters for their children:

> We are recommending and asking for a mandate that allows parents, along with the advice and counseling of their doctors, to make a decision regarding their own child. If a retardate is being cared for in the home by parents, they should be given the right to make a decision regarding their own son or daughter. We feel that we as parents, are intuitive and realistic and in the best position to recommend either a tubal ligation, a hysterectomy or a vasectomy; the latter to prevent any chance of false accusation of paternity.[33]

Parents' groups not only played an important, and vocal, role in these debates but also introduced additional elements for consideration. Parents voiced concerns about reproduction, and about the care of potential grandchildren, with a lingering subtext concerning the likelihood that such children may also exhibit intellectual or physical disabilities. In addition to these issues though, disabled daughters posed a different set of challenges than sons, and parents explored hysterectomies as a method of ending menstruation for women who required personal care. In one case, parents considered sterilizing their fourteen-year-old daughter after determining that she was incapable of taking care of her own menses. In that instance, "they felt it their duty as caring parents to relieve her of the discomfort of menstrual periods and proceeded to arrange for a hysterectomy."[34] In this example, the parents had already consulted a doctor, who agreed that the operation would benefit the young woman as well as her parents. The parents, however, sought additional legal protection, adding that "most of these girls are going to have periods and they are going to talk about them and (if [name removed] had a hysterectomy) she is going to be different. The kid may be madder than hell at her mother in three or four years time."[35] The parents' group further examined alternatives, speculating that putting their daughters on the Pill for more than thirty years seemed unreasonable, and they questioned its long-term reliability. They posed the question directly: "With the new Family Reform Act now in effect making parents responsible for children and grandchildren, are we as parents going to be held responsible for the rearing of another child, possibly a retarded one?"[36] Responding chiefly to fears of transmission and menstrual hygiene, parents sought legal protection.

Zarfas intervened by demanding that the CMPA provide guidance to physicians working with institutionalized populations, after newspaper headlines warned that doctors could be charged or at risk of losing their licences for breaking this law.[37] Zarfas stepped back from the individual cases and commented on concerns about physician liability. Discussions continued to hinge on protecting doctors from legal repercussions, more so than any concern for the well-being or autonomy of individuals being subjected to sterilization.

Zarfas's views on parents were informed by a survey he conducted with parents of children with disabilities about their attitudes toward birth control in southwestern Ontario. He contacted three hundred parents in Essex, Middlesex, and Waterloo Counties to gauge their

reactions to birth control for their disabled children, shifting the focus
away from mental disorders or intellectual disabilities to questions
of hygiene for individuals who were physically disabled. His preliminary report showed that parents overwhelmingly supported sterilization in the form of tubal ligations, vasectomies, or hysterectomies
(67 per cent) over other options, including no birth control (12 per
cent) and contraceptives including the Pill, IUD, condom, or injectable
long-acting birth control (16 per cent).[38] In spite of these views, only
7 per cent of the parents interviewed had sterilized their children,
while 69 per cent relied on supervision from a combination of parents
and professionals. The discrepancy in the numbers suggests that
parents were keen to have their children sterilized but encountered
difficulties in procuring the service. The *Hamilton Spectator* published some of the results of this study under the headline "Parents
of retarded favor sterilization," explaining to readers that 71 per cent
of parents interviewed "strongly favoured sterilization without consent
in cases where the child was declared incompetent to decide."[39]
Zarfas's study reveals that regardless of the sex of the child, parents
sought and even anticipated involuntary sterilization as a necessary
part of their children's care plan and, indeed, as a consequence of care
in the community.

The CMPA at this time stated emphatically that doctors should not
initiate discussions about sterilizations but rather should allow parents
of patients to make requests for such operations. In a sustained effort
to avoid future legal challenges, the CMPA recommended a thorough
set of assessments by a variety of medical professionals, including
family physicians, psychologists, psychiatrists, and possibly social
workers, to ensure that any decision about sterilization had sufficient
documented professional support to stand up to legal scrutiny.[40]
Building upon past legal precedents, Zarfas stated that the procedure
in all cases should be explained to the child before proceeding,
if all other parties were in agreement. His language – describing
people with disabilities as "children" – further infantilized individuals
who fell into this category, reinforcing the idea that they required
protection from a paternalistic state with laws designed to make
decisions on behalf of dependent children or adults and their families.
Moreover, those decisions should rest on the shoulders of parents and
not physicians, according to the CMPA.

Ultimately, the CMPA, together with the Ontario Medical Association, established a set of guidelines for assessing the conditions for

sterilizations. After convening a special committee on children's health services, the joint committee of legal and medical advisers recommended that sterilizations of people considered mentally retarded, of either sex and of any age, could proceed if there was "clear benefit to the patient," if "there was clear evidence of existing risk of pregnancy" drawn from evidence that might include "evidence of heterosexual experimentation," and if the patient was considered fertile but where other means of contraception were deemed unsatisfactory.[41] The directions and guidelines stipulated by the CMPA reflected its familiarity with the challenges posed by the Alberta eugenics program and its legacy in the 1970s, particularly of its lack of consent considerations, which ran roughshod over patients who had been deemed mentally incapable of providing it: "We are particularly concerned about anything which might appear as an established program for 'wholesale' sterilizations of these patients ... We would be particularly concerned about the sterilization of a child unless the operation were requested by interested, concerned and attentive parents."[42] Whether responding to provincial sterilization policy or historical examples as extreme as those in Nazi Germany, the legal advice doled out to physicians by this time stressed the need for consent as a sacrosanct feature of modern medical interventions – but this time, consent from parents. Parents, according to the CMPA, could make informed decisions about their children's sexual and reproductive lives that struck a balance between individual rights and individual protection. This approach also reflected older ideas of girls and women as virtuous and in need of protection from sexual predators – a perception that had applied more broadly to all women in public discourse of the 1920s. In the 1970s these same concerns were amplified in the context of deinstitutionalized populations, with the fear that women in particular would be subjected to increased degrees of sexual abuse.

Even with guidelines in place, hospitals and sterilization boards struggled to interpret them, which frustrated parents. In February 1979 the *Globe and Mail* reported that a hospital had refused to sterilize an eleven-year-old girl with Down syndrome, against the direct wishes of her parents. The parents expressed their outrage at not being consulted about their daughter's future; her case was determined by a sterilization committee consisting of a psychiatrist, pediatrician, psychologist, social worker, hospital trustee, school principal, and housewife.[43] Zarfas responded to the parents, suggesting that women with Down syndrome had quite an expansive set of abilities, and parenting was not out of the question. Zarfas then borrowed phrasing from the parents' commission, suggesting that this girl may become "madder than hell" later in life upon learning of the consequences of a hysterectomy.[44]

DISABILITY AND DEPENDENT ADULTS

The Law Reform Commission of Canada had concluded by the end of the 1970s that individuals with mental illnesses "should not be sterilized against their will." Indeed, stated the LRCC, mentally handicapped persons "should have the same rights as other persons to consent to or refuse sterilization as long as they can understand the nature and consequences of the operation."[45] Provinces, however, had developed their own guidelines regarding sexual sterilization and abortion operations for residents of their institutions. Alberta's Dependent Adults Act introduced different approaches to identifying and obtaining informed consent by elevating third-party decision-makers and fundamentally triangulating the politics of choice as it concerned reproductive autonomy of those deemed incapable of deciding for themselves.[46] This assembly of decision-makers resembled the composition of eugenics boards, in effect extending the tradition of a relationship between psychiatric and custodial institutions and eugenics. Working in direct contrast with the CMPA, the law commission in Alberta instead looked to clinical professionals to make choices on behalf of institutionalized or recently deinstitutionalized patients of childbearing age. Several of the people who had worked in the institutions now filled those positions in the community but retained ideas about sexuality and deinstitutionalized people living in the community.[47]

Donald Zarfas also supported this recommendation, in part because it took the decision-making away from parents. He based his interpretation on a series of surveys he had made of parent perspectives. For instance, in 1979 he requested permission from the Ontario government to examine "the attitudes of parents who have retarded children to try to understand their level of sophistication in the sexuality of their offspring and what their attitudes are in relation to the concept of sterilization." It was already clear to Zarfas that the Ontario Association for the Mentally Retarded had issued statements in opposition to sterilization; he noted that the president had "expressed herself as being vehemently against sterilization and this, in itself, may bias the sample from which that opinion is collected."[48] By expanding the survey to all parents of children considered intellectually or physically disabled, Zarfas hoped to generate a clearer case for decision-making that did not rely solely on parents. Some might have gone further, to argue that genetic risks outweighed environmental concerns. The context of civil rights for deinstitutionalized patients, therefore, complicated the discourse of liberty and autonomy as a paternalistic approach that persisted when it came to this population.

Zarfas emerged as a controversial figure in these debates, as he promoted sterilization as a feature of (ex-)patient liberty that went hand in hand with the struggle to close institutions and allow people to live semi- or fully independently in regular society. He acknowledged that having children was a privilege, not a right, and moreover that the privilege was becoming even more significant in "this over populated world."[49] Addressing the Ontario Psychiatric Association in 1978, he stated that the rising tide of rights-based movements around the world

has brought about the recognition of rights for retarded persons, whether they live at home, in community residences or in institutions. The recognition of their rights to an education, to treatment, to protection from abuse, to the due process of law, and, ultimately, to the right of life, has a tremendous effect on the retarded's place in society today ... [T]he retarded must be seen as individuals and not as a class of subhuman and inferior beings. We must give recognition to the retarded's right to self-determination within reason and his right to protection from abuse, even if we appear to be acting in his best interests.[50]

Walking a fine line between protection and restriction, Zarfas attempted to articulate the need to both humanize and protect this segment of the population. He later went on to insist that individuals had a right to sexuality and sexual expression, yet he identified sterilization as a vehicle for achieving this liberty. In other words, Zarfas implied that people living outside of institutions and back in the community, with or without intellectual disabilities, should have access to the same reproductive and sexual health services, including sterilization as a form of birth control. In this regard, the suggestion positioned women with intellectual disabilities on an equal footing with middle-class feminists who had lobbied for sterilizations as a form of birth control.

These kinds of awkward alliances or convenient bedfellows have been a mainstay in the history of eugenics. American historian Johanna Schoen, for example, illustrates how the politics of race and ability routinely complicated campaigns for birth control. For white women with resources, a campaign revolved around the choice to have children, while for many other women, especially impoverished and racialized women, access to healthcare services was already lacking and a long tradition of racist and sexist policies led many to distrust the medical establishment when it came to matters of reproductive health.[51] A similar narrative unfolded in Canada surrounding Indigenous women whose access to health services had languished behind those of their non-Indigenous counterparts. The decision to give birth in hospitals, and subsequently be sterilized, or to remain at home without proper prenatal, antenatal, or contraceptive care presented women with very different contexts in which to exercise their so-called reproductive choices, as described in chapter 2.

The overlap between coercive eugenic sterilizations and sterilization chosen for birth control continued to complicate the legality of the issue. Zarfas made this point explicitly in a plea to the OMA: "I am certainly not recommending legislation of a Eugenic nature. I am recommending, however, legislation that will provide the protection we have suggested so that incompetent people may have the right to enjoy the benefits of sterilization as do myriads of their competent peers."[52] Extending elements of protection from the state into arguments for individual freedom, Zarfas borrowed from the discourse of social movements that helped to justify the need for continued professional surveillance over former institutionalized patients, who were implicitly women, making decisions about their reproductive lives.

In one revealing paper on the sterilization of "mentally retarded females," Zarfas wrote, "Let us immediately state that we are only dealing with the sterilization of mentally retarded females, because, whatever her condition may be, there will always be a male ready to copulate and impregnate this defenceless being." He added, "It was never found difficult to decide that they should have an appendectomy or dental treatments. Since it is very obvious that they cannot take care of a child because they cannot even take care of themselves, the decision to sterilize them should not be so difficult unless fertility is still regarded in name as an unmitigated blessing for everybody, which it is definitely not." He further explained that sterilization is preferable to contraception, as it "is run only once."[53] Much like his contemporaries across Canada and the United States working in the field of "mental retardation," Zarfas emphasized the language of burden, irresponsibility, and health risks associated with leaving these individuals unsterilized. In other words, the logical humanitarian response, according to Zarfas, was to sterilize these women so that they could live freely and safely, without fear of becoming pregnant. Implicit in this discussion is an extension of rights-based logic to a group of people lacking the same rights and services that would allow for such a free choice in the first place. Moreover, many of the women he was describing continued to live in institutional or quasi-institutional settings. Despite efforts to promote an ethos of care in the community, Zarfas and others working in the system quickly recognized that many of the people leaving institutions were not reuniting with loving families but instead shifting into halfway homes and other facilities, where they may be vulnerable to abuse and certainly were not expected to thrive independently with the kind of freedom of movement or independence afforded to most of mainstream society.

INSTITUTIONAL VERSUS MENTAL HYGIENE

After the 1969 Criminal Code amendments, it is unclear whether women in the community were taking advantage of their newfound sexual freedom or not, but within institutions the concerns about fertility went beyond those associated with pregnancy. One of the focal points of this discussion was the matter of personal hygiene. In fact, one such case, involving a mother trying to have her daughter sterilized to alleviate her menstruation, reached the Supreme Court of Canada in 1986.[54]

Eve was a twenty-four-year-old Prince Edward Islander with "extreme expressive aphasia" – that is, a difficulty in speaking – and limited learning abilities. During the week she was institutionalized in a facility for people with "mental disabilities" and on the weekends she lived with her mother, Mrs E. According to hospital administrators, Eve began developing an interest in one of the male residents, who was also described as disabled, and they informed her mother. Mrs E felt that her daughter did not appreciate the concept of marriage and could not be responsible for raising a child; ultimately, she requested that Eve be declared mentally incompetent under the provisions of the provincial Mental Health Act. Following that designation, Mrs E suggested that she should be given the power of "substitute decision-maker" and that Eve be sterilized for nontherapeutic reasons. The case bounced through the court system, beginning in a provincial family court and ultimately landing in the Supreme Court, where the country's highest judicial power ruled against Mrs E's request and set a new precedent in the country for denying the role of third-party or substitute decision-makers in sterilization cases for people considered mentally incompetent. The timing of the *Eve* case was significant. The decision, in 1986, came shortly after the introduction of the Canadian Charter of Rights and Freedoms (1982) and preceded other common law jurisdictions that were similarly struggling to find the legal balance between *parens patriae* and individual rights. In many cases, the state was also reconciling the legacy of eugenics, which further complicated discussions about who could make decisions on behalf of people considered mentally incompetent. This point was made even more significant in an era of deinstitutionalization or psychiatric care in the community, as the dynamic concepts of prevention, protection, and individual rights were being reevaluated and redefined.[55]

Eve's case was not an isolated incident but served to widen the public discourse on this topic. In Calgary, an administrator at the Grace Hospital explained that he had experienced three recent cases of female minors who were considered incompetent, incapable of controlling their bodily functions, and "unable to look after their personal hygiene."[56] The parents in each of these three cases had requested hysterectomies for their daughters when they reached puberty, anticipating the challenges of dealing with their menses. Once again, Dr Zarfas was called upon to comment on the case. Here he also agreed with the logic behind this reasoning even while disagreeing with the right of parents to initiate the requests. He argued that sterilization was justified "where hysterectomy is contemplated for control of menstruation in a seriously-retarded person, all measures to train the child in management of menstrual discharge by competent professional trainers have been unsuccessful, and oral or parenteral contraceptive steroids are either unsuccessful or not tolerated." He went on to state, "It would be possible for an emancipated, retarded youth to give consent; however, one must be certain that this patient knows the nature and consequence of the surgery. One should also be assured that external coercion is not forcing the decision."[57]

Zarfas's arguments rested upon an assumption that a return to the community involved a return to parental control for most of the individuals who had been living in custodial institutions. Given that the parents he had surveyed held strong views in favour of sterilization, a return to the community did not mean relinquishing the institutional control over one's body; rather, it formalized the triangular decision-making over children's and dependent adults' reproductive bodies. The situation thus retained rather than removed the arguments for preventing procreation by people considered mentally or physically dependent, or in need of supported care, and thus deemed them incapable of producing independent and healthy children.

Across the country during the 1970s, animated debates raged over consent and contests took place over who has the authority to determine whether a dependent child or adult was a candidate for sexual sterilization. In Ontario, parents continued to press for surgeries for their dependents. Health minister Dennis Timbrell had spoken against the practice, but it became clear that parents were resorting to other means, including travelling to other jurisdictions, to secure the operations. Much like women who travelled for abortions to circumvent constrictive legal provisions or service obstacles, some parents took control of the situation by leaving the province.[58] In 1979, OHIP reported paying for 126 such operations, including hysterectomies, tubal ligations, and vasectomies, despite existing prohibitions. Given these findings, the OMA recommended lifting the moratorium on sterilizations for dependent children but supported the creation of an oversight committee that would consider whether such an operation was "in the patient's best interest."[59] It appeared that people seeking sterilization, whether for themselves or for their dependents, were willing to go to drastic lengths to secure the surgeries but that physicians remained uncomfortable relinquishing the decision entirely to parents.

It was not until 1982, with the introduction of the Charter of Rights and Freedoms, that individual choice became more formally enshrined in the legal landscape. The context of the 1970s, therefore, involved a murky legal territory for teasing apart the relationship between the state and the individual in contests over who decides whether one is capable of responsible parenthood and how that debate trickles down to regulate an individual's fertility. The debates over reproductive health and access to health services remained pregnant with protectionist, even paternalistic, discourse when it came to people considered physically disabled, mentally ill, or intellectually delayed. Not all reproductive bodies laid claim to the same degree of "equal" citizenship rights in practice, yet the language of rights continued to frame debates over how best to accommodate all Canadians.

In 1986, the Supreme Court's decision on *Eve* drew a decisive line in these debates. The ruling revealed that despite past justifications for seeking nonconsensual sterilization – whether to prevent pregnancy, reduce long-term care costs, or control menstruation – neither the state nor families had a role to play in recommending this surgery. The legal reports that followed spelled out a new era for sterilization in the mental health arena: "With *Eve*, the ground rules have completely changed. Concern about the potential for unwarranted sterilization of vulnerable individuals has been replaced by concerns about a situation in which those not competent to legally give their consent are barred from access to this form of birth control or menstrual management. The message 'we will not let you risk having babies' of the eugenic sterilization days has changed to the message 'we insist that you risk having babies.'"[60]

The *Eve* decision represented a significant shift away from preventing people considered mentally incompetent from reproducing and toward preventing an abuse of power over these people, by denying sterilization surgeries for all people declared incompetent under mental health laws. Questions of mental health and competency continued to function like a hinge in these decisions, swinging the door open to sterilization for nearly half a century and then swinging it in the other direction as a declaration of mental incompetency became a reason for restricting sterilization under any circumstances. These decisions run precisely opposite to the rationale used for so-called healthy or competent members of society, who were denied access to contraception until 1969 and then increasingly embraced it as a feature of modern human rights discourse. By 1988, the Canadian figures matched those of other western countries, showing that sterilization had become one of the leading means of contraception: nearly 70 per cent of women used contraceptives, including sterilization surgery. The Commission on Sterilization Decisions reported that 68.4 per cent of Canadian women of childbearing age used some form of contraceptive, and 35 per cent of those women had chosen sterilization; another 12.7 per cent had a male partner who had had a vasectomy.[61] These numbers suggest that sterilization had become a significant form of birth control in Canada by the end of the twentieth century.

CONCLUSION

Major custodial institutions began emptying in the 1960s and 1970s, ushering in an era of deinstitutionalization, and the idea of reintegrating their former residents into communities gave many people pause. Patients' rights movements merged comfortably with other human rights rhetoric that embraced the language of liberty and autonomy as a basic tenet of individual rights; however, despite the rhetoric of patients' rights, patients and ex-patients did not always get to enjoy the liberties that came along with the promised claims.[62] Patients and ex-patients continued to be targeted for sterilization in the 1970s, while the legal parameters were furnished with new justifications to uphold the tradition of forcing certain individuals to undergo procedures that undermined their autonomy. The mental hygiene movements of the 1920s had referred to the pressing need to rid society of allegedly undesirable citizens: those who, because of heredity, character, poverty, or lowered intelligence, threatened to destabilize progress. Half a century later, the language was updated to suit the culture of rights that permeated the 1960s and 1970s, but the underlying assumptions about preventing disorder and disability remained intact.

At the end of the 1970s, personal hygiene replaced mental hygiene as a reason for sterilization. The focus also shifted back to women as those most in need of hygienic intervention and fertility control. It remains unclear as to whether the women targeted by these interventions appreciated the shift in justification, but the results remained fixed: sterilization of these women continued and even became part of the landscape of care in the community. The shift was replete with a human rights agenda suggesting that controlling reproduction within the population contributed to a reduction in the number of people suffering from psychiatric and intellectual disorders.

CHAPTER FIVE

Vasectomies and the Dilemma of Male Reproduction

In 1976 Alvin Ratz Kaufman, a ninety-one-year-old industrialist and Kitchener, Ontario, millionaire, was honoured as a pioneer of birth control by Planned Parenthood in Ontario. Hailed as a philanthropist and visionary for a lifetime of distributing birth control information and devices and arranging for surgical sterilizations through his Parents' Information Bureau, Kaufman was the respectable elder statesman of the new politics of reproduction. Planned Parenthood invited Kaufman to present a brief to the Ontario provincial cabinet on the best methods for distributing birth control information in hard-to-reach northern communities. This invitation acknowledged that Kaufman's methods for distributing birth control technology and information had been effective for several decades, despite the illegality of the practice throughout most of his life.

The timing of this celebration is significant. Even a few years earlier, sterilization was routinely associated with coercion, especially through its association with eugenics. But that connection had been dramatically reframed, such that individuals like Kaufman, who may have at one time been criticized for subscribing to eugenic views, were now being celebrated for those same ideas. Indeed, Kaufman never wavered from his firmly held eugenic motivations, which he had honed during the Depression. Although he was careful in presenting these views publicly, his approach remained consistent. His eugenic, and financial, interest in birth control interventions has received some attention from historians who have focused especially on how he pedalled this information through his female employees and even created incentives for birth control use among his factory workers.[1] His approach to male sterilization and support for vasectomies, however, has not garnered the same attention. In fact, Kaufman emerges in this history as a somewhat emblematic and distinctive figure. Much of the history on eugenics and birth controllers in the early part of the twentieth century centres around female reformers, such as early eugenicists Margaret Sanger, Dr Helen MacMurchy, and Emily Murphy, who have factored in this history as uncomfortable heroines – or complicated villains, depending on one's interpretation. Feminists have more often been at the centre of this story, having not only lobbied for access to birth control but also promoted restrictions on fertility for women in lower classes or from non-Anglo and nonwhite backgrounds.[2] Kaufman's participation in these debates suggests that men were also directly involved in these earlier campaigns, but his motivations likely differed from the feminist claims made by women like Sanger or Murphy. Few would accuse Kaufman of being a feminist, but his elite social status and decades-long commitment to facilitating access to birth control made him an appealing figurehead among 1970s birth control activists. Yet, as will be seen, his role in this history is also significant for the emphasis he placed on vasectomies and male birth control.

VASECTOMIES IN THE HISTORY
OF BIRTH CONTROL

The history of vasectomies in the 1970s presents an intriguing case of contradictions. Male sterilization rarely garnered mainstream attention during much of the twentieth century, either in a sustained way in the public discourse or, later, in historical scholarship. Sarah Shropshire's article on vasectomies in Canada sets it in a North American context to argue that changing constructions of masculinity in the postwar period made vasectomy increasingly popular, yet Canadian men were comparatively slow to embrace the operation.[3] Vasectomies, like female sterilizations, had been part of eugenics programs, such that in some jurisdictions vasectomy became a means to parole. California, for example, maintained a policy that some male prisoners could seek parole if they had served their time and were willing to undergo a vasectomy.[4] The association between vasectomy and criminal behaviour served to forge a connection between vasectomy and coercion, eugenics, and discipline. Recipients of vasectomies in this context were those who had transgressed the law or failed to live up to expectations of responsible citizens. Yet, Kaufman

avoided falling into this category with his recommendation of vasectomies. Instead, he placed vasectomies on par with female birth control
measures, aligning himself with fellow activists in the swelling ranks
of Planned Parenthood who, by the 1970s, were readily presenting
the vasectomy as a virtuous act of responsibility. In other words,
choosing a vasectomy represented (under this logic) a selfless act, a
courageous decision to help save the environment by not contributing
to population growth, and, of course, the greatest gift a man could
give his wife.

The vasectomy underwent a character reformation not unlike female
sterilization during this decade, but it did not require, or indeed inspire,
a popular movement to arrive at this reconceptualization. In this way,
the social history of vasectomies is quite different from that of tubal
ligations or hysterectomies. Historically, women were victims of coercive sterilization, but throughout the twentieth century, women had
also been vocal advocates of birth control, especially as control over
reproduction fused with other features of women's political and economic status as citizens. Men had actively participated in these debates
about women's bodies, tending to claim that female physiology prevented women from taking an active role in politics or high-paying
professions.[5] They had remained comparatively silent on how male
physiology translated into power or responsibility. Also, men did not
form a corollary world view to feminism, nor did they need to invent
a "masculinism" to challenge a hegemonic power structure; the male
body was seemingly inherent to the existing hegemonic power structure. Reconceptualizing the vasectomy as a progressive or responsible
choice for the modern man therefore relied on a different kind of
struggle for recognition than that faced by women.

The spectre of population control created an opportunity to con-
ceptualize male fertility without necessarily relinquishing power or
acknowledging that a focus on reproduction represented weakness
in men, as it did for women. Instead, the focus on controlling fertility
was about taking responsibility for the planet and improving economic
and environmental circumstances for future generations. While the
connection to the earth's future may have remained rather abstract
for many men, the idea provided a coherent internal logic that contributed to the reconceptualization of vasectomies. Beyond those
men who underwent vasectomies as part of an institutional program,
whether in jails or in mental hospitals, the majority of men choosing
vasectomies in the 1960s and 1970s were white, well-educated

professionals, middle- and upper-class fathers with means, doing their part for the economy. Vasectomy did not imperil this particular group's claims to hegemonic masculinity, which is equated with and defined by power and portrayed through "whiteness, wealth, education, intelligence, attractiveness, strength, athleticism, fatherhood and heterosexual prowess."[6] Vasectomized fathers maintained, and indeed enhanced, their manhood by representing their choice as serving others' needs, whether their wives' health, their families' economic position, or the world's future. Amid shifting definitions of masculinity and fatherhood in the post–World War II period, the breadwinner role took on a more urban and suburban domesticity focused on family consumption.[7] Taking control through vasectomy protected the family's economic future by limiting family size. Vasectomized men, reassured that their sexual prowess would be undiminished and with their procreative powers proven, could redefine their masculinity around the familiar themes of power, control, strength, and bravery.[8]

A.R. KAUFMAN AND THE PARENTS' INFORMATION BUREAU

Kaufman appears in this moment as one of the few Canadian men who had long been vocal about vasectomies and who, to some extent, championed the procedure as a reflection of male responsibility, albeit directed more locally to working-class families. Kaufman's own role fits the pattern of contradictions in this history. As a capitalist, Kaufman's own reasons for promoting male vasectomies seem to have had more to do with his bottom line and his frustration with the lack of attention paid by working-class families to rampant fertility. He worried that taxpayers were supporting the under- and unemployed families who were too indolent or lazy to take responsibility for themselves. Yet, as he was being feted in 1976, the logic of contraception had changed, from birth control aimed at the so-called underclasses to birth control for the professional class as a badge of civility, honour, and modernity. To some extent, for the middle classes, the shifting conceptualization of male sterilization mirrored female sterilization as both men and women embraced the procedure as liberating, and a performance of responsibility. It is not clear in the records whether sterilization abuse haunted racialized men and boys as it did women and girls, but vasectomy continues to be a more popular form of birth control for middle-class men than for working-class men.[9]

The comparative silence on male birth control during this period reminds us that many of these discussions took place in the shadows, in contradistinction to discourses of women and birth control at the same time. It is a reminder too that redefining the value of the vasectomy involved different discussions of power, responsibility, and control.

Vasectomy – where the male vas deferens is cut and tied or sealed to prevent sperm from entering into the urethra – is a quick, simple, and effective method of surgical sterilization. Like tubal ligation for women, it has emerged from its long association with eugenics to become a popular form of permanent contraception.[10] However, the similarities all but end there. By the 1970s, as an inexpensive and simple procedure that could be performed in a doctor's office, vasectomy attracted less public attention than tubal ligation, which until then had involved major abdominal surgery requiring general anesthetic, several days in hospital, and a lengthy period of recuperation. By contrast, a vasectomy required only about twenty minutes, a needle to the scrotum to deliver local anesthetic, some pain from the incisions, a day or two to recover, and of course a cooperative physician. Until 1971, the group that insured doctors, the Canadian Medical Protective Association, had advised that surgical sterilization was illegal unless performed for the preservation of life – a difficult argument to make in regard to vasectomy – but the privacy of a doctor's office shielded the procedure from oversight. After 1971, the CMPA relaxed its position on male surgeries, drawing vasectomies more in line with voluntary sterilization for women. For women, hospitals maintained pronatalist age/parity rules such as the "120 formula" (a woman's age multiplied by the number of her children had to equal 120 to allow for her surgical sterilization), though physicians still wielded considerable autonomy, as we have seen. Dr W.J. Hannah, a Toronto obstetrician, explained that sympathetic physicians who agreed to provide a tubal ligation "invoked sometimes genuine, more often imagined physical disabilities" that might jeopardize a women's life if she had any more pregnancies. One of the most common indications for the operation was the presence of varicose veins.[11] No such hospital procedures or administrative policies governed physicians who chose to provide vasectomy.

Into the 1970s Kaufman's Parents' Information Bureau maintained a list of "cooperating" physicians to whom Kaufman might refer men who inquired about vasectomy. His interest in birth control and sterilization had begun in 1929 when his laid-off workers at the Kaufman Rubber Company complained that they had families to support. As Kaufman put it, "I asked the nurse to check on the home conditions ... [S]ome of the mothers were more or less mentally deficient and poor housekeepers. I asked the nurse to suggest sterilization to the fathers in order to prevent having more children; but I expected contemptuous refusal. I was surprised and somewhat embarrassed when my suggestion was welcomed." Kaufman sent a "sympathetic" doctor, his cousin Dr Ratz, to visit the Margaret Sanger Clinic in New York to learn about surgical contraception procedures: "He returned and sterilized a few men who, with their wives, evidently lacked sufficient motivation to use contraceptives consistently."[12] As author Linda Revie notes, it is probable that some of Kaufman's workers were retained on the condition that they underwent vasectomy.[13] Indeed, he had a fraught relationship with his employees at Kaufman Rubber and his nearby Superior Box plant, a paper box making factory. Patriarchal and "tight-fisted," Kaufman faced down the United Rubber Workers in a 1937 strike that ended after two weeks; Kaufman locked his workers out for another month to discourage unionization. Again in 1960, bitter and violent strikes at his plants resulted from years of intimidation and union busting.[14] Kaufman's personal eugenics campaign targeted what he called the "welfare classes," the poor and unemployed whose large families drained the resources of members of the "tax paying classes" like himself. He was an executive member of the Eugenics Society of Canada (established in 1930) and brought along his cousin Dr Ratz and local physician J.E. Hagmeier, co-owner with Kaufman of nearby Preston Springs Sanatorium and Clinic.[15]

By 1968, Hagmeier (then aged eighty-four and still active) had vasectomized over one thousand men referred by Kaufman, who also provided operating facilities at his rubber factory for local doctors who performed multiple vasectomies in succession.[16] Prospective vasectomy patients completed PIB application forms and, if approved, the bureau enlisted the services of a willing physician near the patient's home – but it was Kaufman or a nurse who mediated access to the procedure. As long-serving nurse Anna Weber explained, in one case, a man from Saskatchewan who applied for vasectomy was not "considered a suitable one for sterilization as they [the couple] seem to be intelligent, therefore should be capable of controlling pregnancies through the use of contraceptives ... [W]e exercise great care when selecting them as we are primarily interested in the needy and the most incompetent."[17] The dependent and "sub-normal" needed sterilization, according to Kaufman, who claimed, "Personally, I think they ought to be dumped in the lake."[18]

The PIB's clandestine work connected Kaufman with a larger international network of like-minded eugenicists, especially the Human Betterment Association of America (HBAA) in New York. Indeed, as the HBAA executive director wrote to Kaufman, "Our aim is to rival the acceptance which you have achieved in Canada."[19] Kaufman continued to make annual financial donations to this eugenic association after it changed its name to the Association for Voluntary Sterilization (AVS) in 1965. As Kluchin argues, the AVS maintained its eugenic motivations but changed its tactics: "Their new goal was to convince the poor and unfit to voluntarily terminate their fertility; their agenda became less about preventing the 'unfit' from reproducing and more about helping the 'unfit' poor to limit their family size and improve the quality of American citizens this way."[20] The AVS referred inquiries from Canadians to the PIB and Kaufman reciprocated, while the groups shared lists of willing physicians who would perform vasectomies.

Kaufman shared the AVS's motivation to limit the reproduction of the poor and unemployed, but he was increasingly out of step with the organization's changing tactics. In the late 1960s, the AVS adopted the rhetoric of the population controllers who feared a population explosion as the preeminent threat to national and international security and saw the need for sterilization to meet that threat.[21] Kaufman, however, remained firmly convinced that social welfare agencies should require parents of families receiving their services to use contraceptives or be sterilized. He never tired of boasting of his successes during the Depression when PIB social workers dispensed contraceptives to "nearly 100,000 homes of poverty stricken parents." Forty years later he continued to equate the poor with crime and depravity: "Unwanted and deprived children are potential rebels and criminals in a society that has too many now. How can we expect to reduce the crime rate when the highest birth rate is in these classes?"[22] For Kaufman, sterilization was essentially punitive. As he told John Rague, executive director of AVS, in 1966, prisoners who agreed to a vasectomy should be offered a six-month reduction in their jail sentence. Furthermore, he suggested that the legal punishment for rape should be vasectomy on the first offence and castration on the second offence. A prisoner should forfeit his fecundity "since society does not want more of his type."[23] Kaufman continued to advocate forced sterilizations, while the AVS maintained that "the voluntary acceptance of sterilizations in the US and around the world would diminish if there were any forced sterilizations."[24] Kaufman in many ways represents a more typical proponent of eugenics, particularly as evidenced by his vocal disdain for people considered feebleminded, underemployed, or within the margins of criminality. The fact that he continued to promote vasectomies into the 1970s is a poignant indication of how quickly public attitudes were changing with respect to this surgery that continued to linger in the shadows, both in terms of discourse and in clinical encounters.

Vasectomy occupied a legal grey area in the United States and Canada before the 1970s, and opposition from organized medicine forced the PIB and AVS to maintain discretion. But during the 1960s, as public discussion of sex and sexuality became more acceptable, print media brought vasectomy out of the shadows. A 1960 article about surgical sterilization in *True Story*, an American magazine in the "true confessions" genre, led to fifteen inquiries to the PIB; Kaufman arranged for ten vasectomies but refused three as "unjustified."[25] A 1961 article in *Maclean's*, a Canadian news and general interest magazine, generated attention well beyond the PIB's expectations and more than seven hundred vasectomy inquiries. The article, titled "The safe, certain birth-control method that doctors won't talk about," compared vasectomy to having a tooth pulled by a dentist, but with rather less pain: "Vasectomy cuts off the flow of sperm – the male fertilizing agent – but has no other physical effect on the man's sexual system."[26] With obvious input from Kaufman, the article estimated that two hundred men had undergone the operation in that year, with the help of the PIB, "a private organization … devoted to giving advice about birth control." Echoing Kaufman's frequent outbursts in his correspondence regarding the malign motives of organized medicine, the article blamed the Canadian Medical Association for keeping vasectomy from Canadians. Men seeking vasectomy were characterized as desperate, if not heroic, in their efforts to protect their wives from dangerous pregnancies. It noted that the anonymous "Dr. Zed, a handsome, athletic father of three children," had performed his own vasectomy when no physician would agree to do so. This pseudonymous doctor was clearly Donald Dodds, a Toronto physician who performed two vasectomies a week on patients referred and screened by the PIB. Dr Zed was one of only six doctors (three in Vancouver, one in Edmonton, and one in Kitchener) in Canada willing to cooperate with the PIB. Readers were told that the operation was safe, it was inexpensive, and there was no actual law forbidding it. But one man's experience, having travelled to the United States for a vasectomy, reassured readers where it counted the most: "One thing really had me worried. I wondered if I'd ever be the same again – I mean sexually. I had read that the operation has no effect whatever on a man's sex drive and that the only thing that changed was his ability to father children. My worries proved needless. Married life now is even more satisfying and pleasant than it's ever been, probably because my wife and I know we're off the hook of constant parenthood forever." Frank discussions of male sexuality were rare in the mainstream media, and the news of a simple inexpensive operation that leaves men with their manliness and even improves their sex life was sure to generate interest. Readers were also reassured that vasectomy would likely be reversible in the near future. According to a follow-up article, in the fifteen months since the first article had appeared, the PIB had received one thousand requests for vasectomy.[27]

In a 1963 *Chatelaine* article, "Vasectomy: How one couple ended the fear of dangerous pregnancies," Larry Ross recounted how, after six "wonderful children" in thirteen years of marriage, he and his wife had reached their economic and emotional limit. A chance meeting with a "Toronto doctor" who recommended vasectomy directed Ross to the PIB. He noted, "I prefer that people seeking sterilization discuss the matter with this bureau first, due to their extensive work in the field of family planning and related problems." Ross articulated his fears around the loss of fertility: "I am not so sure of myself on a psychological plane. I shrink from the idea of having someone tamper with my manhood and I suppose I have some irrational fears of castration." The surgery was simple and successful. A year later, Ross reported that his wife's health had improved and that he had no regrets, as "both the mental and physical aspects of our sexual union have become more rewarding."[28] This magazine article presented vasectomy as a reasonable, rational choice for middle-class men who sought to protect their family's economic, physical, and emotional well-being.

The article generated 110 inquiries in ten days at the PIB, though Kaufman estimated there would be five times that number in total. Of course, those inquiring needed to be screened to ensure they were suitable candidates for the surgery. A man with a large family was by definition suitable, because he was clearly too incompetent to use contraceptives. If patients could not afford the fee, the PIB paid physicians a twenty-five-dollar honorarium. Increased publicity created a demand for vasectomies that tested the PIB's ability to mediate access to the procedure; Kaufman and his nurse could only hope that poor and "unfit" people were among the growing numbers choosing vasectomy because they needed it most: "We find that about 90% of the better class applicants have the vasectomies completed, while the shrinkage in regard to the less intelligent may be 50%. We can judge the caliber of the applicants by the caliber of the magazine."[29] Even the rather staid CBC Television program *Close-Up* took an interest, with a 1962 episode featuring birth control opponents, including the editor of Montreal's *Le Devoir* newspaper and advocates Barbara Cadbury, Dorothea Ferguson (née Palmer, Kaufman's employee charged in the 1937 PIB nurse trial), and Kaufman himself, who denied the charge of manufacturing contraceptive devices in his rubber plant and who claimed that his "arithmetic wasn't good enough" to calculate the financial cost of his philanthropy in service of birth control.[30] Kaufman regretted that TV broadcasts failed to generate the same interest in contraception as print media.[31]

THE ECONOMICS OF VASECTOMIES

Surging interest in vasectomy after positive media reports highlighted the bottleneck in the PIB's operations. With only twelve sympathetic physicians who would provide vasectomies, Kaufman relied on the Human Betterment Association's referrals in border areas, but he had no access to physicians in the Maritimes, southern Saskatchewan, or Manitoba. In July 1962, he hoped to entice Saskatchewan doctors who were on strike against that province's health insurance program, though his lawyer cautioned against sending out circulars requesting cooperation for fear of antagonizing medical associations.[32] By the end of the decade Kaufman claimed that the PIB had referred almost four thousand applications for vasectomy to cooperative doctors since 1963 and that at least ten thousand vasectomies had been carried out independently in Canada.[33] As he noted, vasectomies had once been a great secret, but with open discussion in the media and among men in their own networks who referred their friends to cooperative physicians, the PIB became superfluous.

Still, Kaufman pointed out, there remained those in the "welfare classes" who did not know enough to choose vasectomy. Social welfare organizations repeatedly refused his offers of assistance to promote birth control among their clients. So, in December 1969, the PIB placed an ad in the local Kitchener newspaper offering free contraceptives and sterilization of parents receiving welfare. Kaufman recalled, "We did not get even one inquiry in 15 months; but the ad started a flood of inquiries about Vasectomy from people who stated they were not on welfare and quite willing to pay ... Evidently the poor do not read the papers to any extent or take any initiative."34 Kaufman, to his great disappointment, stumbled upon the phenomenon that the academic literature was also documenting: that vasectomy was increasingly popular among white, middle- to upper-class men. This shift was precisely what was driving the popularity of the vasectomy, but it was also redefining the procedure as a tool of individual responsibility as opposed to collective irresponsibility.

If men were reticent about discussing vasectomies in public, women were less reserved. One 1968 article in the *Globe and Mail* boldly asserted that "women should stop struggling with contraceptives and instead force men to submit to sterilization through vasectomies."35 Also in 1968, the *Globe and Mail* described Ellen Verwey, a Vancouver-based sociologist, as an "ardent feminist" who at the noted age of fifty-two addressed the Royal Commission on the Status of Women with the suggestion that men should bear more responsibility for birth control, and moreover, that the vasectomy operation was simpler, cheaper, and more easily reversible. The newspaper also reported that Mrs Verwey, as she was identified, held a Ph.D. in sociology, she was married with no children, and her husband had first-hand experience with the operation. The problem, however, according to leading urologists, was not Verwey's contention that vasectomies could be reversed – they agreed that approximately 60 per cent were successfully reversed – but rather that the law did not permit physicians to perform these operations "because it is not helping the male patient's health." According to urologist Dr John Balfour, "In the case of a woman, it is different because we are doing something for her health in preventing pregnancy. It is a fine distinction, but it does exist." Verwey disagreed. She suggested men did not seek vasectomies out of "male selfishness." She explained that "men preferred to force women, the subservient sex, to take precautions that could prove dangerous to them." Women take hormonal pills, they engage in risky abortions, all to prevent pregnancy, sometimes taking their own lives into their hands. The unnamed reporter went on: "Mrs Verwey, a short, square woman with dark hair, said that in India men who have had three children are persuaded to have vasectomies by an incentive system. 'You can get a transistor radio by agreeing to one.'"[36] Despite the off-putting, and rather insulting, ways that Dr Ellen Verwey was described in this report, she was not alone in advocating for the male vasectomy as a more efficient and practical way to promote birth control, alongside women's liberation. But the reception to her article, and indeed the tone of the report itself, underscores how the issue was not one of finding male allies for a feminist campaign; rather, vasectomies were shrouded in their own discourse of responsibility.

The economics of vasectomy were difficult to deny and perhaps provided an easier point of entry for the discussion among some men. A year earlier, the Ontario Medical Association had approved the principle of voluntary male sterilization. The CMPA, however, disagreed with this move and refused to provide insurance or cover malpractice suits associated with vasectomy operations. The OMA explained that "large numbers" of men were now seeking the procedure, billed at $85 per operation, compared with $150 for a woman's tubal ligation. If men wanted this operation, the OMA reasoned, why should it not be provided?[37]

Vasectomy quickly became a cultural phenomenon. The *Toronto Star* in 1974 declared that "vasectomy is now 'in,'" commenting on the radical change from a time when women had almost always assumed responsibility for birth control. Canadian and American men sported gold and blue enamel lapel pins that bore the letter "V" for vasectomy. British men wore ties featuring a stylized "V." Advertising their most "personal and intimate bit of medical history," the pins and ties also assured women (accurately or not) that "you won't get pregnant by me."[38] But vasectomy was seen almost exclusively as a decision made by couples. Most physicians continued to require the consent of both partners, and few would sterilize young, childless, and/or single men.[39] The numbers were impressive (and increasingly reliable as physicians claimed the costs from provincial Medicare plans): 30,000 vasectomies in Ontario in 1974. Dr Donald Dodds performed 6,500 vasectomies in Toronto; Oakville's Dr Ross Prince performed 3,500; Vancouver's Dr Philip Alderman over 3,500; and two doctors in London, Ontario, sterilized 8,000 men. The publicity would not have harmed the physicians' booming practices while prospective patients were comforted knowing they would be in experienced, and steady, hands.

The *Star* dismissed recent research that had linked vasectomy to decreased hormone production and increased risks of arthritis, rheumatic fever, and multiple sclerosis; it also dismissed men's fear that vasectomy would undermine their masculinity. Indeed, wives reported improvement in their sex lives: "Since Ted's operation, sex for us has become spontaneous and free. I can get completely involved with my husband." A Toronto doctor advised that it was in fact the man with the large family who exhibited grave doubts about his own masculinity, having previously handled his inadequacies by keeping his wife pregnant.[40] A sociological study of eight hundred men who underwent vasectomies in London, Ontario, in the late 1960s, noted the increasing popularity of the operation and pointed out that, historically, birth control techniques (coitus interruptus and the condom) had been male oriented. It was only in the twentieth century, and with the more recent focus on women's rights, that pessaries, creams, jellies, the IUD, and the Pill had come to dominate birth control. Men's former dominant role in family planning had been challenged by women, but with vasectomy men were reasserting the "traditional values and norms of western society." The rise in the incidence of vasectomy was a "male backlash" to the feminist movement, the authors argued; "males, realizing the weapon women have over them when reproduction is under female control are beginning to reassert themselves." These modern men, husbands, were the "innovators"; they were from the professional and managerial rather than semiskilled classes, with wives (median age of thirty-three) who had ten to fifteen more childbearing years, and all of the men undergoing the procedure already had more children than they desired.[41] But, as Dr Edward Shapiro of Ottawa told Planned Parenthood volunteers, physicians should still decide who ought to be sterilized. He warned that both partners needed counselling on the physical and emotional effects of a vasectomy: "I have often refused a vasectomy and urged the woman to have a tuballigation because she was better equipped to handle it. Vasectomy is a great operation for the right man, but it is a disaster for the wrong man."[42]

VASECTOMIES AND POPULATION CONTROL

In the *Toronto Star*, George and Barbara Pratt talked about their decision to have a vasectomy. Under a photo of the couple happily playing with their sons, aged three and six, the Pratts admitted that their decision was a personal one: "Two children are enough. There are other things in life besides babies and diapers." The story portrays the Pratts as a normal, rational, and healthy Canadian family. George, a sales manager, who lost just one day of work for the operation, could continue to support the family financially. Barbara, a former schoolteacher, had no plans to return to work. Joining the conversation was Dr Marion Powell of the Population Unit at the University of Toronto's School of Hygiene, who pointed to population control as evidence that the Pratts had made the responsible choice. "Far from fanatics," the Pratts knew about Zero Population Growth and other groups that warned of the dangers of the population explosion not just in Asia but in Canada's overcrowded cities. Population controllers lauded greater awareness and adoption of birth control measures, but as we have seen, this was often directed at perceived "problem" populations. As Barbara Pratt admitted, the couple had faced some criticism of their decision that George would have a vasectomy: "They said we're well off and could afford more kids, that we're intelligent and that we're good parents." Critics argued that if Canada had a population problem, it was that there were not *more* Pratts.[43]

Other influential critics worried that men were being unduly pressured to undergo vasectomy for the wrong reasons. Columbia University researchers David and Helen Wolfers called the efforts by population controllers and propagandists in the press "vasectomania," arguing that vasectomy had "the uncanny knack of gathering enthusiastic support from the fringes of the medical profession and the public." Their brief survey of its history appeared to bear that out, as vasectomy went from being a procedure to cure masturbators to a weapon for eugenicists, then offered purported benefits for sexual rejuvenation, and finally was heralded as a means to avert a population explosion and global disaster. Men, Wolfers and Wolfers argued, should never be told that vasectomy is the greatest gift they can give to their wives, or that their libido will increase, or that vasectomy is usually reversible, or that it might help solve the world's problems. Men should never be pressured, "however light or subtle" the pressure, to undergo vasectomy; it should be his decision alone – a decision that is free, unprompted, and informed. Young men lured into vasectomy, they wrote, "will live deeply to regret the mutilation of their bodies, their severance from the mainstream of human life, and the lost opportunities for love and fulfillment in the long life ahead," thereby ending up "a bitter bank of outcasts, disqualified from the joys and responsibilities of normal men by an hour's surrender to the voice of the death wish."[44] So-called vasectomania highlighted some of the excesses that accompanied shifting contraceptive technologies, but it also took for granted that men (unlike women) had an inherent right to bodily integrity and reproductive autonomy that needed constant protection from changing social and medical understandings of sexuality. Masculinity needed vigilance so that men, given the unbiased facts, could be free to make their own choices while women, feminists and wives, were conspicuous by their absence.

Vasectomy, an intimate medical procedure, had a way of making the news. A 1977 *Globe and Mail* article, "Vasectomy: Gaining Fast in the Birth-Control Race," was typical of a genre of personal testimonials that were considered newsworthy.[45] Reporter David Lancashire wrote, colourfully, that "it's a nervous man who clambers on to the table and feels the quick jab of a needle in the scrotum as the doctor injects the anesthetic, like a dentist freezing a tooth. After that, he feels nothing. The doctor stands between the patient's legs, cutting away a fraction of the vas deferens ... and knotting the ends with silk thread, working with the deft nonchalance of a housewife sewing on a button."[46] It seems no detail was too personal to include – in contrast with vasectomy's otherwise shadowy existence in private doctors' offices. The reporter's characterization of the surgical procedure resulting in a loss of fertility as a wifely domestic task aimed to normalize vasectomy as a rational choice for the modern man and, in particular, "a better bet than the Pill." To that end, the article visited vasectomy's progressive history, from the early days, when Kaufman's concerns for the unemployed led him to advocate birth control and sterilization, to heroic Dr Donald Dodds describing, again, how he performed his own vasectomy when no other doctor would do it. Vasectomy was increasingly popular, according to the *Globe* article, which reported 25,998 vasectomies "last year in Ontario alone."[47] (As we have seen, three years previously the *Toronto Star* reported 30,000 vasectomies in Ontario.) In fact, vasectomy was losing badly in Ontario's birth control race: the vasectomy rate was still less than half the rate of tubal ligations.[48] Nevertheless, vasectomy testimonials presented narratives of masculine stoicism, constraint, and pioneering bravery. Dr Robert McClure, medical missionary and former moderator of the United Church of Canada, recalled his own vasectomy in 1933, done in China: "I had done two or three major operations at the Anglican mission hospital and I climbed on the table and the other doctors did me. Then I climbed down, did a couple more operations, put my knapsack on my back and walked six miles to the railway station."[49]

The reporting on vasectomy in the medical literature, particularly large-scale studies, tended to emphasize the procedure's benefits rather than its side effects. As the Wolferses noted, reports of postoperative increases in sexual prowess and coital frequency were "waved aloft like ball game scores."[50] Mass vasectomy camps in India, where nearly seven million men were operated on in return for cash payments, had no equivalent in the West. Still, by the time Dodds gave up his practice in 1976, he claimed, he had performed 7,613 vasectomies.[51] Calgary's E.S. Livingstone impressed readers of the *Canadian Medical Association Journal* with his report of performing 3,200 vasectomies over eleven years. He described the incidence of postoperative complications lessening over time as his technique improved. Only one of his patients became impotent after the operation, "but it was learned from his wife that impotence had been present intermittently for some years before."[52] Livingstone advised using local anesthesia for its convenience and economy, since no anesthetist was required, because patients could return to work more quickly and, interestingly, because it demonstrated the minor nature of the procedure, "so that those who desire it are not deterred." Livingstone's large study group ranged from a twenty-one-year-old "low intelligence epileptic" to a seventy-five-year-old, with an average age between thirty-five and forty. He noted that all occupations were represented, "with the exception of long-term welfare cases which were conspicuous by their absence." The frequency of vasectomy, he found, increased among groups of men who worked closely together; 30 to 40 per cent of a group of firefighters had had the operation, while at one station all the men were vasectomized. Homosocial environments that included both work and domestic space, such as a (1970s) firehall, add to our understanding of the links between vasectomy and the performance of masculinity.[53]

Apologizing for his study's comparatively small size, Edmonton physician Michael Richards reported in 1973 on his series of 296 vasectomies – a number that "may appear insignificant." Richards justified its inclusion in the medical literature by his noteworthy technique. He vasectomized unmarried men only reluctantly, because it would abrogate their human rights, but otherwise there were few contra-indications. Richards relied on the Parents' Information Bureau consent form, signed by the patient and his consort, "if there is one." Key to the procedure, for Richards, was to relax the patient: to engage him in conversation on any subject of interest to him "and let him talk!" Relaxed and distracted, patients were surprised when the quick and simple procedure was over, at which point Richards, in full view of the patient, placed the resected vas in jars that were then sealed and signed by the patient. The sealed jars were kept in the office as a medical record. Richards's collection of "sealed jar evidence" protected him against accusations by women that that the operation had been a failure because a wife "(or friend)" became pregnant. Richards explained that this was "borne out by personal experiences as a witness in divorce proceedings and a paternity suit."[54]

The reported side effects remained minimal while, over time, word got out that the benefits were significant. It turned out that women enjoyed sex more when the fear of pregnancy was removed. Although the public discussion continued to centre around married, heterosexual couples confronting these new realities, the language of relief coupled with the pride of responsibility made the vasectomy a heroic option, and wives became obliging supporters. In this way the language of responsibility associated with the vasectomy did not need to compete with feminism for control over fertility but could more comfortably sidle into the conversation on its own terms. Some feminists may have bristled at how celebrating vasectomies allowed men to reap social benefits and recognition without having to confront the deeper inequalities that divided the sexes, but at least for a moment in time, the ends justified the means. By the end of the decade, vasectomy was firmly a feature on the progressive landscape.

Nowhere was the uptake more dramatic than in Quebec. Historians have noted that the Quiet Revolution in Quebec – historically characterized as the most Catholic of the provinces – coincided with a contraceptive revolution. Quebeckers eagerly embraced contraception in the 1960s and 1970s. American data suggests that in the 1970s over eleven million people, roughly divided evenly between the sexes, underwent a sexual sterilization procedure. In Quebec, between 1971 and 1978 the rate of vasectomy nearly doubled, from 5.5 per 1,000 men (aged twenty to forty-nine) to 10.0 per 1,000, the highest in the country.[55]

In the same time frame, women's tubal ligation rates rose from 4.4 per 1,000 women (aged fifteen to forty-four) to 21.1 per 1,000, or double the male rate. This dramatic uptake in elective sterilization procedures indicates a strong correlation between access and acceptance of the procedure as safe, effective, and perhaps even a necessary feature of modern life.[56] In their comparative study social scientists Nicole Marcil-Gratton and Evelyne Lapierre-Adamcyk speculated that differences in healthcare systems may explain the differential uptake by the sexes in the United States and Canada. Since the male procedure was cheaper, more American men might be willing to undergo that procedure rather than have their wives seek out the more expensive tubal ligation. In Quebec, as elsewhere in Canada, both procedures were covered under Medicare, suggesting that concerns about responsibility continued to linger.

Vasectomy increased in popularity across Canada through the 1970s and 1980s. Initial surges in 1971 and 1972 saw vasectomy rates equal to or greater than tubal ligation rates in Alberta, British Columbia, Saskatchewan, and Quebec.[57] This likely reflected the relatively easier access to vasectomy than to hospital-based tubal ligation; it may also have been the result of pent-up demand. By mid-decade, national tubal ligation rates (18.1 per 1,000) were more than double the vasectomy rates (6.9 per 1,000), though the differentials between the two rates steadily narrowed for the next decade. By 1986 the rate of vasectomy had increased nearly 40 per cent, while the tubal ligation rate had decreased by 27 per cent. Important regional differences remained. By the 1980s, more vasectomies than tubal ligations were performed in Newfoundland, while in Quebec men and women were sterilized at the same rate. Quebec's vasectomy rate (12.2 per 1,000) was double that of neighbouring New Brunswick (6.4 per 1,000).[58] Regional differences are not easily explained, but access to providers may have been a factor. A 1982 study concluded that personal choice was likely the reason more women than men underwent sterilization: "In many couples, the choice as to which partner will have surgery is made because one partner will not consider being sterilized, and this partner is twice as likely to be the husband."[59] In most regions, this was an obvious conclusion.

In Vancouver, Dr Philip Alderman was the "expert's expert." Associated with the PIB, he began performing vasectomies in 1965 and, by 1974, had performed 3,500 operations.[60] Among his vasectomy patients were 47 of his medical colleagues, both general practitioners and specialists. Alderman reported the reasons his physician-patients chose vasectomy over their wives' tubal ligation: safety, economy, and convenience. These particular experiences were also valuable for providing testimonies that might help to describe the advantages of a vasectomy to inquiring patients.[61] By 1988 Alderman had given up his practice as a family physician to specialize solely on vasectomies. Not a disinterested advocate, he and his coauthor Ellen Gee advised health insurance policy makers that the cost advantage of vasectomy (about $75) over female sterilization (about $133) should recommend its greater use. They noted that in 1974 in the United States the rates were roughly equal, though tubal ligations were on the increase; in Canada, though, the differences between male and female sterilization rates were narrowing, and some regions showed the opposite trend. Alderman and Gee recommended that professional health and family planning counsellors actively promote vasectomy.[62]

Indeed, in 2009 in Canada vasectomy was twice as common as tubal ligation. Canada was and remains one of only five countries in the world where male sterilization is more common than female sterilization.[63] But sharp regional and class differences emerged. A 2013 study in Manitoba found that vasectomy rates were highest among high-income (southern) residents, while tubal ligation rates were highest among lower-income (northern) groups. The association of vasectomy with social and economic advantage had frustrated Kaufman and the eugenicists, and it persists. The lower invasiveness and physical risks of vasectomy appear to be reserved for the most advantaged. The study's conclusions may reflect differences across classes in decision-making power and responsibility regarding reproductive health or differences in access to health care.[64]

CONCLUSION

The politics of reproduction were recalibrated when it came to vasectomy. As the mechanics of the operation became a topic of public discussion, coupled with the discourse on global fertility and both public and individual responsibility for advancing modern civilization, vasectomies emerged from the shadows and joined the conversation. The topic did not merely merge into ongoing conversations about feminism or reproductive rights, however; it entered on its own terms and relied on its own vocabulary to describe the significance of vasectomy in modern life. If women could now enter the workforce in greater numbers and in a wider diversity of positions because they could plan their pregnancies, men could set their sights on global economic developments because their vasectomies allowed them to perform an act of national or even international responsibility. While this rhetoric may have helped to animate the discussions, or even to tip the legal scales of justice toward relaxing laws on access to vasectomies, the empirical evidence suggests that men were participating in this reconceptualizing process. Professional and middle-class men may have initially shared tips about which doctors to see, or what to do for a quick recovery, or even how the procedure affects one's sex life or notions of masculinity. They may have conducted these conversations on the golf course, reinforcing the idea that such chatter took place in private. But within a decade the rates of vasectomy use had climbed significantly. Men and women overcame any lingering fears about moral damnation, and concerns about physiological damage subsided relatively quickly, especially as techniques became better understood and more openly discussed.

In the end, both men and women participated in this reframing. And, as in the case of abortions and female sterilization, the spectre of population control helped to galvanize support for the decriminalization of and increased accessibility to vasectomy. Whether population control was something that was happening in the Global South or among working-class families in southern Ontario, the idea that birth control, including vasectomies, could lower the birthrate appealed across a wide spectrum, uniting for a moment those who subscribed to the language of individual autonomy as well as those who lobbied for more collective responsibility. In this precarious moment, before the emergence of HIV/AIDS once again altered the tone of the conversation, vasectomies were part of a responsible approach to managing modernity.

CHAPTER SIX

Teenagers and the Economics of Abortion

The partial decriminalization of abortion in 1969 by the federal government was a bittersweet victory for women. The issue attracted considerable media and public attention. Some felt that legalizing abortion, even under restrictive conditions, spelled certain disaster for the moral sanctity of Canadian families. Others felt that the laws had not gone far enough in safeguarding women's choices and capacity to secure a surgical abortion without first surrendering to the increasingly controversial therapeutic abortion committee. The public debate also refocused the moral discussion of irresponsible parenthood onto young women.

Pregnant teenage girls emerged in this period as the most alarming category of individuals seeking abortions. Their youth and (predominantly) unmarried status signalled sexual promiscuity and fuelled anti-abortionists' claims that such operations merely contributed to the moral and social decay ushered in by liberal reforms. On the one hand, some Canadians appeared upset by the possibility of "abortions on demand," which they associated with irresponsible middle-class feminists who challenged traditional family values. As described in chapter 1, parliamentarians tended to side with physicians and chose to impose the TACS on women seeking abortions. This additional barrier and layer of judgment meant that in cases of teenage pregnancy, the pregnant woman or couple were rarely the only ones involved in making decisions about family planning. On the other hand, some of the key players in these debates, whether physicians or policy makers, appeared less conflicted about proceeding with abortions, in combination with or separate from tubal ligations, on women and teenage girls for whom they believed parenthood presented serious challenges.

This chapter examines some of the responses to teenage abortions across Canada and analyzes how feminists participated in a shifting discourse on choice when it came to minors.

TEEN PREGNANCY EPIDEMIC

Concerns about an "epidemic" of teenage pregnancies spilled through newspapers and captured the attention of Canadian physicians. Debates on the topic spiralled through news media, into local high schools, and through Planned Parenthood Organizations. In reality it was not clear whether teens were increasingly engaging in sex, but the cultural context had changed sufficiently with the expansion of a welfare state that allegedly provided a greater set of services aimed at protecting Canadian families, even those headed by young single mothers. As historians Karen Balcom and Karen Dubinsky have shown us, the prospect of single motherhood and rising rates of teen pregnancy in the 1970s also animated conversations about adoption, including the premise that children were being rescued by white, middle-class families.[1] Adoptions across cultural lines also produced cross-border adoptions, as both Balcom and Dubinsky explore in their studies of how adoption patterns revealed deeper attitudes about nation-building priorities and merged with family planning discourses.

Among much else, the so-called sexual revolution of the 1960s had also unleashed an era of sexual experimentation that seemed to accept premarital sex. Megan Blair argues that for unmarried women, accessing birth control or abortion services presented significant challenges. She examines how student activists at southern Ontario universities organized to lobby for better sex education that included explicit guidance on birth control, sexual health services, and abortion.[2] For many Canadian parents, teachers, guidance counsellors, and others who did not identify with sexual liberation, teens remained ill informed about sex and especially about contraception. Whether Canadians teens actually participated in unprotected sexual intercourse in increased numbers remains debatable, but Statistics Canada began reporting an increase in the number of babies being born to teen mothers. Even more worrying was the fact that more teen mothers than ever before were keeping their children.

In 1982 the *Canadian Medical Association Journal* featured a special report on the topic in an attempt to weigh in on the public panic about teenage sex, referred to as "babies having babies."[3] The article suggested that the number of teen mothers was in fact declining, but this decline was due in large part to the increased reliance on therapeutic abortion services. However, viewing data over the entirety of the 1970s, the authors surmised that Canadian teens – contrary to their British and American counterparts – may in fact have been having less sex and using more or better contraceptives. Furthermore, the authors suggested that women in particular now had more options to consider: "In the past, women who became pregnant when unmarried either got married or put the baby up for adoption. They now have two other options: they can have an abortion, or remain single and keep the baby, often with the assistance from social welfare agencies and the government."[4] They concluded that as a result of these newly available services, fewer young, single, pregnant women were putting children up for adoption, which in turn was giving rise to a perception of a "crisis": that teenagers were increasingly raising children on their own. The authors explained, however, that the perception that more teenagers were becoming pregnant was in fact false, based merely on the increased visibility of pregnant teenagers. Generations earlier, women who had become pregnant out of wedlock were more likely to conceal their condition by moving to homes for unwed mothers, or relocating to other communities for the duration of the pregnancy, after which point the children were sometimes adopted formally or informally, such as by relatives. In reality, fewer teens were becoming pregnant, but those who did were choosing to either abort or keep their babies. Despite the explanation these authors provided in the CMAJ, Canadians continued to worry about the fate of teenagers in the context of shifting legal and moral terrain on abortion.

COUNTING ABORTIONS

Statistics Canada paid close attention to the age and marital status of women having therapeutic abortions and began reporting on abortions in annual reports starting in 1972. Without a clear baseline for measuring the numbers of abortions, the reports give an impression of rising requests for abortions and a growing array of reasons that women presented to justify their need for an abortion. By 1975 these reports included a separate section devoted to teenage abortions and marital status.[5] From that point on, the number of abortions for teenage women increased: from 15,447 in 1975, to 16,731 in 1976, and 17,719 in 1977. The vast majority (95 per cent) of these teenagers were unmarried.[6] By 1977, Statistics Canada claimed, over 30 per cent of the abortions performed in Canada were for women under twenty years of age; of those cases, 14 per cent were fifteen years of age or younger, 38 per cent were sixteen or seventeen, and the remaining 48 per cent were eighteen or nineteen.[7] For the vast majority of these teenagers, the abortion represented their first pregnancy.[8] The distinction between abortions for married women, usually over the age of twenty-five, and single women, more often under twenty-five and, increasingly, under twenty, framed the responses by government, not-for-profit, and anti-abortion activists alike as they attempted to redefine the moral terrain on abortion, reproductive choice, and feminine morality in the wake of the legal changes.

These national statistics quickly supplied empirical data suggesting that teenagers were securing abortions. Rates of requests were also rising among the unmarried under-twenty age group, making some reformers uncomfortable about how abortion services were being used and what this might mean for the future of Canadian families. While medical complications were possible in all age groups, statistics showed that "the abortion complication rate was highest (7.6%) for women under 15 years of age."[9] And with 16,731 therapeutic abortions provided to women under twenty in 1976, the potential for serious complications was not insignificant.[10] The focus on teenagers and young women might have stemmed from a genuine concern for the welfare of these women but may also have emphasized the risks to help dissuade unmarried teenagers from seeking abortions, or from pregnancy in the first place. Reports from the early 1970s paid particular attention to younger cohorts. Over the period from 1974 to 1980, the therapeutic abortion rate per 1,000 females was highest for women between twenty and twenty-nine (12 to 16 per cent) and women under twenty (9 to 13 per cent). By comparison, the rate for thirty- to thirty-nine-year-olds was 6 to 7 per cent, and for those over thirty-nine it was 2 to 3 per cent.[11]

Age arose as an important factor not just in terms of securing abortions but also in terms of risk – including emotional distress, regret, and physical damage to one's reproductive organs – and associated surgeries to prevent pregnancy. Some women sought sterilization at the same time that they had abortions. The majority of requests in this category came from married women who already had children. Statistics Canada reported that, in 1975, "about 50% of the abortions with concurrent sterilization were between 25 and 34 years of age, another about 40% between 35 and 44 years of age, accounting for close to 90% of the sterilized cases for all age groups."[12] Additionally, "more than 71% of sterilized cases had between one to three previous deliveries and another about 23% had four or more previous deliveries."[13] Resultantly, older women were much more likely to have concurrent sterilizations than were younger women. Of those women sterilized in 1976, most had had previous deliveries: "More than 73% of the concurrently sterilized cases had between one to three previous deliveries and more than 21% of the cases had at least four previous deliveries."[14] These figures suggest that despite the rhetoric that teenage abortions presented more risk, most sterilizations were occurring among married women between the ages of twenty-five and thirty-five, many of whom already had children. Whether these statistics more accurately indicate how Canadian women applied for abortions or how TACS responded to such requests remains unclear because of the paucity of available and accessible medical records. Nonetheless, teenage pregnancies did not fit into a model of family planning considered acceptable, primarily owing to age and marital status.

After 1969, Statistics Canada began tracking the number of abortions performed in each province, ultimately demonstrating that the numbers of these operations rose dramatically over the first ten years, even as provinces and hospitals scrambled to put the services into effect. For example, in 1969, only 143 hospitals anywhere in the country reported capacity or willingness to provide abortions. That first year, Statistics Canada reported 4,375 abortions; by 1975 the annual number had risen to 49,311. These numbers are difficult to evaluate evenly, as they also demonstrate not only the slow development of services but also the complicated establishment of TACS that slowed service provision and may have reduced the numbers of abortions. Moreover, the number of teen requests had arisen by this time as an alarming statistic; in 1975, Statistics Canada began tracking this category directly.

While concerns about rising rates of teen abortion requests were no doubt genuine, unmarried teenagers, and single women in general, soon became the predominant subjects of discussions over the new realities surrounding the moral landscape of abortion in Canada. Officials acknowledged that many people were now having sexual encounters before marriage, which they suggested was part of a cultural shift in attitudes, facilitated in part by the increasingly available range of contraceptives. Some scholars have suggested that this moment witnessed the introduction of a "contraceptive mentality," manifested as contraceptives became normalized in the marketplace as well as in sexual encounters.[15]

SEX EDUCATION AND BIRTH CONTROL ADVICE

However, while women in their twenties and thirties appeared to readily adopt birth control, teenagers were comparatively slower to embrace contraception but eager to experiment sexually. It is not entirely clear whether this gap in use reflected ignorance or lingering sensibilities of shame, guilt, or judgment at the drugstore. Karissa Patton's study of sex education in southern Alberta suggests that stigma surrounding premarital sex had profound implications for teens seeking contraception, producing personal feelings of shame or concerns about one's ability to secure employment in a small community where one's reputation could be at stake.[16] Moreover, sex education was sorely lacking. Despite a recognition that teens were engaging in sex, some communities continued to prioritize abstinence and preferred to avoid sex education for fear that it may titillate young students.

Family planners, keen to improve access to abortion services, remained somewhat cautious when it came to teen abortions. Here, family planning associations (FPAs) resurrected neo-Malthusian arguments, suggesting that teenage pregnancy threatened to destabilize populations by creating a generation of children raised in child services or with unstable single mothers whose resources, financially or emotionally, were limited. The fact that Indigenous women more frequently had their children apprehended during the 1960s as part of the Sixties Scoop, regardless of the age of the mother, did not filter into discussions in the mainstream press or in FPAs.[17] Rather than promote female sexuality coupled with reproductive choices, family planners conceptualized teenage girls as a subset of the population that required intervention, protection, and information about how to avoid or terminate pregnancy.

By 1973, Statistics Canada reported that British Columbia had the highest rate of abortions in the country; Ontario and Alberta were tied for second, and Yukon came third.[18] Federal officials quickly surmised that these regions reported higher rates because services were already established in these places on account of their eugenics programs, whereas other provinces and territories were comparatively

behind in developing their abortion services (which does not adequately
explain the high rate of abortion in Yukon). It is worth noting that
in both British Columbia and Alberta, the provincial sexual sterilization acts remained in place until 1973 and 1972, respectively. In
Alberta, the Eugenics Board itself at first doubled as the TAC, thereby
readily providing the infrastructure and government-sanctioned expertise to evaluate abortion requests. The number of Canadians travelling
abroad to get abortions, as Beth Palmer and Christabelle Stethna have
described, also dropped as more services were established in Canada:
20 per cent of abortions for Canadian women were reportedly performed outside of the country in 1969, and just 3.8 per cent in 1976.[19]
So, while these provinces may have had slightly inflated numbers as
women travelled from other provinces to these regions to take advantage of the early adoption of services, the numbers levelled off quickly
and do not sufficiently account for the high number of abortions in
these regions.

Ontario physicians explicitly claimed that abortions were more
dangerous for teenage girls than for older women, and BC government
reports agreed. Medical reports stressed acute as well as long-term
health complications for young women. According to the Statistics
Canada report from 1972, "The mortality rate in teen-age mothers
is higher. Birth complications tend to be greater. The health of the
mother is poorer. The possibility of cervical cancer in later years is
enhanced, and her education and career possibilities are usually
severely circumscribed."[20] Family planners in British Columbia agreed
that the shift in cultural views had ushered in more tolerance toward
teen mothers but also suggested that this relaxation in attitudes did
not sufficiently take into account the health of the mother or the baby:
"Although the stigma attached to out of wedlock pregnancy has
dwindled, and an unplanned baby is no longer considered the 'disgrace' it once was, such a baby has strikes against it in the areas of
physical and emotional security, and its chance for a happy life is
reduced."[21] The report concluded that these findings indicated a pressing need to invest in sex education. The rates of teen abortions seemed
largely to represent ignorance about sexual practices and risks of
pregnancy: "In some centres as much as 20% of induced abortions
are performed on girls under 19 years of age – representing a colossal
failure to educate."[22]

Reports from women's health clinics throughout British Columbia
indicated that they were being overwhelmed by requests from teens
for information and services, which convinced them that more

emphasis needed to be placed on getting resources into schools. As one report indicated,

> An estimated 8,900 patients were seen by clinics in the province in 1972. The largest age group was seventeen year olds with sixteen and eighteen year olds second and third in attendance in the rural and suburban areas. It is interesting to note that approximately one third of patients are new patients and almost 100% are already sexually active, the majority of whom had previously used no birth control methods. This seems an indication that more sex education is necessary in the schools.[23]

Initial attempts at bringing this information into the classroom, however, were rebuffed by parents, who wrote to the BC minister of health, Dennis Cocke, offended that the government appeared to endorse premarital sex by discussing birth control in high schools. Physicians pushed back, arguing that the age of majority (nineteen) created real barriers to providing younger women with abortions or prescriptions for the Pill in that they required permission from their parents, who often refused to comply. Physicians then argued that young women's reproductive options were constrained because these two laws were in conflict. The birth control pill could be dispensed without parental consent for two months, but doctors indicated that after that period teen patients routinely discontinued their use; some doctors interpreted this as proof of their inherent immaturity, while others contended that the need for parental consent for longer-term prescriptions was the real barrier. The province's deputy minister of health identified the problem as generational, suggesting that "an appeal should be made to parents to recognize that society is undergoing a rapid change, even though many of these changes are not acceptable to those from a previous generation. The community is trying to develop ways to cope with these new problems and is in need of active support."[24]

In response to a letter from a woman in Powell River, who had written to the health minister about the need for improving sex education for teenage girls, Cocke wrote,

> As you state, the age of majority is 19 years. It is legal for a person 16 years of age or older to obtain medical advice on their own, and this would include birth control pills. The medical profession is being faced with the problem of children under 16 years of age and it is becoming common practice that where

this child is not living at home, the doctor must provide the medical services which are requested. In this way, the actual practice of treating young children is well ahead of the law and indeed this is the usual custom that the law follows what is actually occurring in society.

He concluded the letter by registering his personal disapproval: "I would like to point out that people from my generation do not necessarily agree with the practices that are occurring among young people today."[25]

The minister remained reluctant to endorse more sex education, but the Vancouver Women's Health Clinic insisted that information about safe sex was not even reaching the high schools at all, in turn creating an undue demand for abortions from young women: "Our contact with younger women has made us aware of the need to communicate our information to students at high schools and colleges ... Almost daily a young woman (14–18 years old) phones for counseling and information regarding termination of her pregnancy. We feel that many traumatic experiences might be avoided if these young women and men fully understood their maturing bodies – physiologically and psychologically."[26]

Desperate to get the message about birth control to teens, in the mid-1970s the FPAS in British Columbia and Alberta adapted an American-based comic book to distribute in Vancouver schools. The comic was produced by Marvel, the publisher of Spiderman, and in fact the same illustrators inked the characters of Joan and Ken Harper in the birth control comic. In it, the Harpers' marriage is in turmoil because they have three children and cannot cope with the thought of another child, but they remain utterly in love, tormented by sexual desire yet repulsed by the thought of another pregnancy. Ultimately, the couple seeks medical help, where they learn about birth control options and, as a result, their marriage is saved. It is unclear how many teens actually related to this adult storyline, though delivered in a teen-friendly medium, but the BC Family Planning Association and both the Calgary and Lethbridge Birth Control Centres purchased hundreds of copies in an effort to better educate young women.[27] The comic did not shy away from the topics of sex and contraception but clearly confined that discussion to the marriage bed.

While most provinces identified particular challenges concerning teen pregnancies, western Canadians, in British Columbia and Alberta,

claimed to have the highest rates. As a result, family planning organizations in these provinces worked to develop specific strategies
addressing the issue: introducing sexual health education in university,
secondary, and primary school curricula; appealing to local governments for funding to support what they defined as a public health
crisis; and tapping into concerns about global population control. At
the forefront of these discussions were family planning organizations
with international connections. These networks of feminists and planners played an important role in defining the so-called crisis in teen
pregnancies and relied strategically on understandings of both feminism and population control in their response to teenage fertility.

Teenage girls fell outside a more mainstream interpretation of
acceptable feminist ideology that viewed reproductive choice as a
critical plank in feminist activism. Teenagers also fell outside of the
range of acceptable independent or autonomous actors according to
government perspectives, which treated teenage girls as a public health
threat who required protection "for their own good"; this, as Cynthia
Comacchio has shown, has a much longer history.[28] In other words,
the politics of abortion access played out differently for these teen
bodies than what we might imagine as a celebration of women's rights
triumphing over a paternalist state. For teenage girls, their choices
were frequently mediated through parents, teachers, public health
officials, and physicians who now overlapped in an effort to place
these girls under sexual surveillance, while leaning on the newly
relaxed abortion laws as a humanitarian option to reduce the number
of allegedly unwanted children.

ABORTION ECONOMICS

Put simply, this process had a lot more in common with the era of
eugenics, where states explicitly managed the fertility of certain
segments of the population, for their own good and for the good
of the population at large. This approach to population control had
deep roots and fused with humanitarian efforts to reduce the individual as well as the collective burden of poverty. The logic had often
extended into particular regions of the globe, most of which were
also targeted for reasons of race and class. A similar argument
emerged in discussions that ostensibly focused on white, even largely
middle-class, urban teens, but in the context of an expensive welfare
state poised to facilitate these life choices in particular segments of

the population where fertility had otherwise historically been encouraged. Teen mothers, more so than teen pregnancies, raised the ante in new ways and reconnected fertility control with a much longer tradition of controlling poverty.

British Columbia, with the highest rate of abortions overall, emphasized education for teens. At the same time, Nova Scotia claimed to have the highest rates of teenage pregnancies through much of the 1970s, describing the issue as a "crisis." The Nova Scotia government, through its Health and Welfare Department, issued a statement in 1978 explaining that the rising rates of teen pregnancy were an assault on modern family values, but the underlying tones were also clear: the crisis was as much economic as anything. The statement asserted that "unwanted pregnancy now costs Nova Scotians a great deal of money and exacts a still higher toll directly chargeable against the stability of the family."[29] Reactions to this claim suggested that "Nova Scotia's teen birth and pregnancy rates are much higher than the Canadian average. Our abortion rate is climbing and is almost certainly an undercount as numbers of Maritime women continue to go to American or Quebec cities for the procedure."[30] Translating those rates into projections, the report indicated that "the sum of total abortions and teen births is rising (and cost over four million dollars in 1978). There is a better than 20% [chance] that any girl turning 15 years old will have been pregnant before her 20th birthday."[31]

Indeed, the spectre of teen pregnancy did not only manifest as a moral issue; government officials were concerned that the rising rates of pregnancy had serious economic consequences: "The girl who has ... a child at the age of 16 suddenly has 90 percent of her life's script written for her. She will probably drop out of school ... [S]he will probably not be able to find a steady job that pays enough ... Her life choices are few, and most of them are bad."[32] This logic continued: "The woman or young couple with an unwanted pregnancy must now stand alone without the backdrop of the extended family and must confront extraordinary financial pressures. The young woman especially stands in jeopardy of forgoing all or part of the education and training she will need to support herself for the rest of her life."[33] It stands to reason that this logic also extended to a moralizing on premarital sex and female virtue, suggesting that a teen mother may not be an eligible wife or partner and that her limited economic opportunities, characterized by both her age and gender, set her on a path of dependency.

While some health officials may well have wanted to avoid circumstances that led teen mothers to become dependent on welfare or social assistance, the concern also convinced family planners and guidance counsellors to invest in specific and targeted education campaigns aimed at teens. These concerns seemed motivated more by concerns over economics than by an interest in the well-being of the teen mothers. Government officials quickly surmised that a new generation of single-mother families had downstream effects on the economy that were at least as significant as the cultural erosion of family values that may or may not result from being raised by a teen mother. These grim prospects convinced health policy makers in the Department of Health and Welfare that investing in abortion services, alongside more aggressive birth control campaigns, would have significant benefits for the provincial economy.

Months after the change in the federal laws on contraception and abortion, Nova Scotia's family planning unit sprang into action. In 1970, the Pictou County Family Planning Association received federal funds to bolster its preexisting voluntary networks and to amplify the public education and counselling services for birth control in rural Nova Scotia. Local concerns about teenage pregnancies in the region had already brought together volunteers who now had a renewed mandate to provide information about sexuality and contraception without risking breaking the law.[34] Their own local research suggested that "most of our sources agreed that virtually all teens who engage in coitus do so without using birth control at some time. It is estimated that a girl has a 16% chance of becoming pregnant during her very first experience."[35] Emphasizing the local conditions, the Pictou County association reported that "in 1951 only 7% of the pregnancies in Canada were adolescents. In 1974, Nova Scotia had the highest rate of teenage pregnancy in Canada, except the Northwest Territories. Today, the probability of a teenager becoming pregnant is over 20%. Approximately one of every six births is to a teenager."[36]

The economic argument was not lost on the family planning organization: "The financial cost to the taxpayer is enormous. It costs, for example, $5,000.00 to the taxpayer for each pound gained by babies in intensive care nurseries. Seventy percent (nationwide) of all children under the care of Social Services are under care due to damage to the central nervous system."[37] They went on, underscoring the cascading challenges of teenage parenting: "In 1974, 50% of births to single women in Canada were to teenagers. For these young women there is a substantial risk of child neglect and abuse. Limited employment opportunities, inadequacy of housing, and lack of emotional maturity are virtually inevitable for the unwed teenage mother. Eighty percent keep their children, rather than giving them up for adoption."[38] These figures were consistent with the claims made in the CMAJ about the rising numbers of teen mothers being the real heart of the problem, instead of the issue of teen pregnancy itself.

In other words, although the rates of teen pregnancy were increasing, the real public policy issue developed out of a concern that, since decriminalization of abortion, more teens were opting to keep their children: "In 1977, 1,625 unwed mothers in Nova Scotia were receiving Social Assistance. This represents a 196% increase over the figure in 1973."[39] Looking beyond national borders, local officials tried to estimate the economic impact of these changes in family structure. Initially, Nova Scotians looked outward for comparators: "In Aberdeen, Scotland a cost/benefit analysis of family planning services was done and a tenfold saving was noted in Health and Welfare over the cost of preventive service."[40] Contraception and abortion services were decidedly more financially appealing than sustained social assistance programs aimed at supporting families, especially when the sole parent lacked education and training due to teenage pregnancy. Pictou County family planners estimated that a reduction of only four social service cases a year would result in sufficient savings to cover the costs of more comprehensive family planning services that aimed at reducing teen motherhood.[41]

Targeting teen pregnancy made good fiscal sense. Investing in family planning in terms of prevention, of both pregnancy and motherhood, created long-term savings to the provincial government that helped to justify a campaign that targeted teenagers. The experiences of teen women who encountered abortion services, however, did not always reflect this reality. It seemed that despite the increasingly convincing financial argument laid out by the Department of Health and Welfare, and pedalled by Nova Scotia's family planning units, teenage girls were still greeted at times with moral arguments about how their actions undermined the Canadian family.

LISTENING TO PREGNANT TEENS

The Halifax Chapter of the Canadian Abortion Rights Action League (CARAL) reviewed the statistics for abortions in Nova Scotia performed in the 1970s and 1980s and questioned why two-thirds of the cases involved single women under the age of twenty-five. In an effort to better understand the reasons for seeking abortions, the local CARAL chapter conducted a series of interviews with women who had passed through the Victoria General Hospital in Halifax, where the majority of these operations took place. The interviews revealed that despite some of the public rhetoric about the problems that teenage girls faced, the women themselves had different views of the abortion procedures. The interviews revealed a variety of the pregnant women's and girls' concerns, from anxiety about wait times to the lack of information or services. The resulting report concluded that each woman "conveyed a strong sense of having endured a difficult experience."[42] However, the commentary went on to state the following:

> Despite the hurt and anger expressed so powerfully by the women interviewed, none expressed regret for the choice she made. Overwhelmingly, they reported feeling relieved once the abortion was over. Some expressed regret that they had ever been in the situation of having an unintended, unwanted pregnancy, but none expressed the wish that she had carried that pregnancy to term. Looking back on their experience, a large majority of the women were able to say that they had come to terms with it, that it had settled satisfactorily into their consciousness as part of their life history.[43]

This admission of feelings of relief, coupled with the dissolution of regret, came through clearly in the post-abortion interviews, yet discussions in the public continued to hold up abortion as a trauma to be avoided by teenagers, in particular.

The women surveyed, many of whom were teens at the time of their interviews, were self selected. All of them were white. Most of them were single. Despite concerted efforts by the research team to recruit women of colour or Indigenous women specifically, none participated in these post-abortion interviews, which may be suggestive of a deeper set of issues related to marginalized women and access to health services or trust of healthcare providers (or perhaps the researchers). As foregoing chapters have demonstrated, the issue of trusting medical professionals has a long and complicated history that may well be reflected also in the willingness to participate in interviews about one's past abortions or decisions to keep children.

The sources are valuable but do not help to address these larger and contentious issues about women's likeliness to talk about abortion in the 1990s when the interviews were collected.

Excerpts from the interviews help to illustrate how women thought of the prospect of pregnancy and its impact on their future. Melissa, from the Halifax Metro area, explained,

> I knew I would [have an abortion] as soon as I found out I was pregnant. I didn't even entertain the thought of carrying the baby, although I guess purely for situational reasons, not reasons that I don't like children, or I don't feel I would be a good mother, not reasons like that. Only because I was only 18, first year of university, I had a lot of plans, and the whole shame thing.[44]

Despite Melissa's relative confidence that having an abortion was her best option, she nonetheless worried about facing a TAC and confessing that she had been irresponsible in having sexual intercourse without fearing the repercussions of pregnancy. She said, "You know, automatically I pictured the board [TAC], and it probably was, as a group of men sitting around and saying, 'What's the matter with this young girl?' And so, I just thought, 'How are they going to know that I really can't do it?'"[45]

Another woman, Stella, explained that her abortion was a rational response to challenging economic circumstances that made expanding her family risky at that time:

> At that time of my life, I just couldn't [carry the pregnancy to term]. It was a really, really bad time, and I don't want to make it sound like a convenience or anything else … I mean, here I was, I was on welfare, had one child … a child having a child, trying to raise him to the best of my ability. Working a little here, a little there, trying to take care of a household, the whole works, everything. And I really, really thought about it. I think I considered every single possibility there ever was … I knew [abortion] was the right decision all along, but I had to admit it to myself.[46]

Arriving at this decision was one step, but convincing the hospital staff that abortion was the best option for her introduced a new set of obstacles. Stella recalled being made to feel irresponsible and unintelligent, which challenged her to reconsider her decision. She

struggled to feel that she was taken seriously by some of the hospital
staff, yet she also described the kindness of the physician who ultimately carried out the procedure: "He [the gynecologist] was just wonderful because he talked to me the whole time he was doing it. He
said that sometimes being talked at while the procedure is happening
makes a person feel much better. It did."[47]

Catharine's experience revealed some of the more gritty realities
and complex factors that affected some young women facing these
choices. Intellectually, she had previously perceived abortion as merely
another health service and one that she would seek out if necessary.
Facing that decision when she became pregnant at seventeen years of
age, however, complicated her feelings about abortion: "Once I was
actually pregnant, though, it was really sort of difficult. Suddenly, it
became very real. I was carrying a child."[48] For Catherine the choice
was further complicated by an abusive partner, who threatened to
cause a miscarriage if she did not abort. She remembered him saying,
"'If you keep this child, I'm going to see to it, as soon as you start to
show, we're going to shove you down a flight of stairs ... I'll do
anything to make you miscarry.' I was definitely scared. I didn't want
to know if he was going to go through with them [the threats] or
not."[49] Taking matters into her own hands, Catherine sought information from *Our Bodies, Ourselves*, a popular feminist handbook on
female sexuality and birth control produced by the Boston Women's
Health Book Collective.[50] Still, she was unprepared for the reality of
the clinical experience:

> The book says that you'll have a nurse there who'll hold your hand
> and be supportive and I didn't get that at the [Victoria General]
> hospital at all ... I knew what the procedure was going to be
> like ... but nothing really prepares you for going into this waiting
> room that's the size of a bathroom and it's filled with 25 people,
> all crammed in, touching each other, knees knocking on the cof-
> fee table ... Completely crammed in there. Nothing really pre-
> pares you for this really mean nurse who is busy saying, "Don't
> scream, don't scream, you're going to scare the other patients."[51]

Another woman recalled that "they treated me like, 'You've been a
naughty girl, and this is what you have to do to make up for it.'"[52]
Feelings of guilt and loneliness resonated in several of the interviews,
as the young women reflected back on their experiences.

Despite the unanimous expressions of relief and gratitude for having had abortions when they faced pregnancy as teenagers, the women nonetheless remembered the shameful feelings and the admonishments from others who suggested they would regret this decision for the rest of their lives. For some, that guilt came packaged in religious belief, with claims that they could no longer face God with a clear conscience. For others, the admonishment came directly from parents who feared their daughters would regret their choices as they later came to grips with their teenage choices and the way they had tampered with fate, or biology, or both. Robin recalled being counselled by her mother to attend a seminar hosted by Birthright, a local pro-life organization. She had argued with her mother, insisting instead, "'I'm having an abortion and that's that.' And they [Birthright counsellors] said 'Oh, you'll change your mind, and if you don't, you'll be *so* sorry. The regret you'll go through in your later years … you'll feel *so* bad.'"[53]

While teenage girls across Canada faced a number of challenges as they sought abortion services, their age and the expectations of their future economic contributions may have also helped secure support for their access to abortions. As one woman put it, after having been asked to explain her reasons for wanting an abortion to the assembled committee, she had said, "Well, what do you mean, what are my reasons? Look at me. I'm just a kid."[54]

ABORTION IN THE PRESS

Public responses to news of rising rates of teenage abortions reinforced a moralizing tone that focused on female virtue. A 1971 article in the *Globe and Mail* lamented the difficulties young women faced in this new era of sexual liberation: specifically, pressure to engage in pre-marital sexual relations, while exposing themselves to increased risks of venereal diseases and the unsettling prospect of abortion. Abortion, according to one Toronto-based physician, left teenage girls depressed and disengaged from mainstream society.[55] While some commentators may have argued that raising a child as a single, and underemploy-able, young woman may equally lead to feelings of depression and despair, the association between regret, depression, and abortion came through clearly in this foreboding article about the difficult pressures young women dealt with when navigating a new era of sexual libera-tion amid a quagmire of risk. Even more damning was a claim in another article by a physician that "one-third of girls who have an abortion during adolescence may find themselves in later life to be anxious, sub-fertile or infertile young wives paying the delayed price for their teen-aged abortion." The article went on to explain that many such abortions also introduce other health complications, some acutely associated with the abortion, including inflammation and infection, and others longer term and more pernicious, such as triggering psychiatric disorders. The article admitted that "both pregnancy and abortion are more difficult and dangerous for adolescents than for mature women."[56] Teen women remained caught when it came to unprotected sex, which for some reinforced the need for teens to engage in abstinence, whereas others argued that the solution was to liberalize access to contraception.

Risks associated with birth control were very real. Despite the popularity of the birth control pill, evidence mounted against its safety throughout the 1960s and 1970s. An American investigation into the safe use of this method of birth control revealed that it had caused damaging side effects for many women, including death.[57] Historian Liz Watkins shows that already in 1961 and 1962 women reported blood clots that had resulted from taking the birth control pill. Within a few years the American Food and Drug Association initiated a full inquiry into the safety of the birth control pill, triggering a set of journalistic headlines exclaiming that the Pill was unsafe and ineffective.[58] Although Planned Parenthood maintained that more women died in childbirth and from illegal abortions, the risks associated with the birth control pill became public fodder for restricting its liberal use.[59]

While some debated the risks associated with the hormone pills, educators maintained that the problem was due not simply to medical technology but to gross ignorance about sexuality and pregnancy. Family physicians in Ontario reported that many of their adolescent patients remained ignorant about safe sexual practices, venereal disease protection, and birth control. Some explicitly blamed Victorian or prudish attitudes held by parents and educators that prevented meaningful conversations about sex from occurring with teenagers before they engaged in intercourse.[60]

Contrary to this logic, however, persistent stigma surrounding teens and sex continued to frame public conversations and may well have discouraged teens from admitting to having sexual relations. Purchasing contraception sent a clear signal of sexual activity. Using contraception, then, became a problem in itself. An October 1972 article in the *Globe and Mail* revealed that, according to an Ontario

Public Health study, the majority of young women who engaged in sex did not use birth control. Of the 175 girls interviewed for the study, many reported difficulties in talking with their doctors about birth control and feared that such conversations would be reported to their parents. Dr Marion Powell, who conducted the study, agreed that the generational differences in attitudes toward sex exacerbated the problem and likely contributed to fewer young women obtaining contraceptives as a result. Consequently, she urged readers to consider the double standard about young women and sex: that sex and sexuality were increasingly on display in advertising campaigns, while young girls were expected to remain chaste and not talk about sexuality. Powell closed by stating that "the major concern is whether serious consequences will develop from this new sexual freedom ... [T]he consequences may be no greater or even less serious than those resulting from growing up in a Victorian atmosphere." She added, however, that "young people will have a lot more fun getting their hang ups than we did."[61]

One BC report summed up the abortion problem as a clash of cultural attitudes with a lack of education about sexual health. On the one hand, the radical liberalizing discourse of free love enticed adolescents to seek hedonistic and self-gratifying experiences, without heeding the consequences, or worse, without knowing the consequences of their actions. The report states, "Sales techniques using sexual symbolism and promoting instant gratification of any desire are adding to the traditional pressures on girls to be popular at any price, and on boys to prove their virility. A combination of ignorance of 'coital gamesmanship' is producing situations such as arose recently in one small northern community where 12% of the junior high school's girls were pregnant at one time."[62] Premarital sex in this context may have provided some social capital within certain circles. On the other hand, teens who crossed this line risked being considered social pariahs in another context, particularly one where they faced parents, teachers, guidance counsellors, or even pharmacists on the topic of sex.

Provinces responded to these concerns differently. British Columbia, for example, in 1965 established a family planning association, an organization run by volunteers, mostly women, that concentrated on providing counselling and education about birth control. Four years later, after the change in the federal law, the FPA was in a position to expand its services and it lobbied the government for direct funds to support its activities. In 1973, the BC FPA organized its first provincial conference around community needs in family planning and involved medical and public leaders in these discussions. At this conference, FPA president Mary F. Bishop, introduced in chapter 3, suggested that the increasingly relaxed attitudes toward sexuality were to be applauded, but that precautions were also necessary to avoid a "crisis – of more and more unwanted and unplanned pregnancies, increasing number of children in the care of child welfare authorities, and an epidemic of venereal disease." She went on to suggest that "the sad consequences of widespread illegal abortion have been solved, to a great extent, by liberalized laws and skilled services; but the demand for pregnancy termination, legal or illegal – like the others, is not so much evidence of new weakening of moral standards as it is of continued lack of rational alternatives in education and prevention."[63]

Bishop explained that of abortions in British Columbia that year, 63 per cent were for unmarried women under the age of twenty-four (35 per cent were for women under twenty), and another five thousand children were moved into the custody of child welfare services, with a later speaker elaborating that these were children born out of wedlock to young mothers. Venereal disease rates among girls aged fifteen to nineteen increased by 11 per cent from 1971 to 1973. These numbers were intended to alarm audience members and rally further support for Bishop's conclusion that more work was to be done to bring sexual health education into the classroom and into public spaces. Now more than ever, Bishop claimed, opposition to birth control was at an all-time low, particularly, as she suggested, because cultural leadership from parents, churches, and police seemed to have waned in significance, which reinforced the need to concentrate efforts on a public service campaign to educate young people about birth control and safe sexual practices. Her claims seem to suggest that because adult attitudes had shifted, they should trickle down to teens.

Conference organizers were pleased with the calibre of the meeting, but ultimately they were preaching to the converted, as no one from government or representing youth organizations – the two key target areas – had participated in the meeting. However, participants did include a variety of Indigenous representatives, from the Union of BC Indian Chiefs to several band councillors. Their participation was important for family planning advocates who also identified Indigenous communities as being in desperate need of fertility control, as outlined in chapter 3. This issue was not lost on local Indigenous leaders.

An article in the *Kainai News*, published on Alberta's Kainai (Blood) reserve, asked whether there was an ideal age for marriage, and how marriage affected family planning: "Many teenagers are also unaware of the opportunities they have. They can only see the immediate future and cannot plan ahead. Maybe because they were not exposed to any other way of life ... or maybe they do not want to because they think they will never meet anyone else. This is where insecurity comes in and restlessness is the result." The article goes on to state that parents should discuss birth control with their teenage children, "educating the child as far as responsibility goes ... [regarding] birth control ... the facts of life ... good ethical responsibility and anything else their child questions."[64] In the case of teenage pregnancy, age and generation seemed to trump race as a category of concern for how to approach sex education.

The BC FPA remained firm in its claims that the global population crisis – that is, the unchecked fertility of populations around the world – was nearing a boiling point. The organization's arguments moved beyond a simplistic Malthusian suggestion that the earth's carrying capacity was being reached, or that food sources were being outstripped by a swelling population, but still reinforced older arguments about the dangerous relationship between poverty and fertility, not to mention age and quality of life.

Canadian delegates from British Columbia attended the United Nations World Population Conference in Bucharest, Romania, in 1974 and brought back with them a desire to link global problems with local challenges of distributing birth control information to young women, Indigenous communities, immigrant communities, and impoverished urban and rural neighbourhoods. Taking a political stance on the need to invoke permanent, irreversible, and cheap population-control measures, these policies revived a much older idea: that poverty and the need for fertility control went hand in hand – and, moreover, that poverty and fertility were two sides of the same coin. Poor people could not be trusted to take care of their reproductive bodies, and their unchecked and allegedly rampant fecundity threatened to destabilize the global economy.

Teenage girls emerged in this context as inherently impoverished, owing to their single status, lack of maturity, insufficient education, and allegedly underdeveloped support networks, leaving them poorly equipped to raise a child independently and especially susceptible to a lifelong dependency on government assistance. The concept of poverty encompassed the anticipated need for publicly funded services in health care, education, and social services, including child welfare services, much of which could be curtailed by investing aggressively in contraception and abortion services for young women. While the government emphasized the poverty of certain women and their families, its concerns stemmed from larger efforts to control public spending in health and welfare services. Instead, it blamed women (and girls) for failing to control their fertility, which then supposedly plunged them into poverty or forced them to rely on the state for lifelong subsistence. The relationship between poverty and fertility continued to be presented, without clear measurements or empirical data to support the association.

Abortions and contraception came to be seen as a key solution to the problem of teenage sexuality and, relatedly, unwanted pregnancy. As indicated in its conference attendance rolls, the FPA regularly reached Indigenous groups, as well as immigrant organizations in Vancouver and throughout British Columbia, but had difficulty convincing the provincial education minister and school principals to distribute information and services within the public school system. More conservative attitudes applied when it came to the spectre of abortion or birth control among young white women and girls. Their alleged promiscuity, and certainly their unwed status as mothers, presented a challenge to family values, but these teenagers could also presumably be protected, or saved, so as to delay their fertility and have families at a more appropriate time in their lives. In this way, birth control and sex education that focused on white teenage girls was quite different than, though inherently related to, the broader global discourse linking poverty and fertility.

For teenage mothers, the risk of succumbing to poverty, becoming dependent on welfare, or losing children to the state became not just an individual concern but one of considerable discussion by policy makers and FPAS. The following explanation is from British Columbia's deputy health minister:

We realize it is a major shock to a parent to find out a daughter is not acting in the manner in which the parent wants her to act. There is an immediate reaction to blame the community service as being wrong and to harm this service by bringing legal action against them ... There is, however, the community side of the problem. This province now has over 10,000 children in care and other children have been adopted in addition. The problem is that these are children who are not wanted by their parents. We know from this information that through habit formation some young girls become sexually permissive. If any attack is going to be made on the problem of young girls becoming pregnant, consideration must be given to preventing the pregnancy, in preference to abortion or having an unwanted child.[65]

According to the deputy minister, parents were a stumbling block to distributing the information necessary for safe sexual encounters and to preserving the image of appropriate family planning. Planned Parenthood organizers agreed with the deputy minister that parents needed to acknowledge that the sexual mores of their generation no longer applied to their children, who faced a different set of cultural attitudes concerning sex.[66]

Yet others tended to place the blame more with the young liberated women whose desire for sexual freedom had not been bridled with the associated responsibilities that come with sex. As one anonymous writer to the BC minister of health described it, "[the] problem has been the recognition of a liberated attitude of women by young girls but without the knowledge to accept the responsibility that goes along with this liberation." Relatedly, this writer offered reasons that teens and young women might not ask their family physician for advice: "either because they cannot take a sexual problem to a family advisor, or because they do not want to let the parents know and a receipt would be sent home from the medical care plan," or because "in some instances, such as travelling youth, the individual did not have medical insurance coverage."[67] Pointing to both structural and cultural impediments, this BC constituent wrote directly to the minister of health appealing to him for joint efforts to resolve the knowledge gap between teenage sexual liberation and responsibility.

MALE RESPONSIBILITY

Interestingly, the discussion at no time centred around men and teenage boys. Men and boys as father figures remained silent and largely invisible in these discussions. Their presence was regularly invoked when it came to providing security, reinforcing a patriarchal set of values that guided the discussion. But, as sexual partners men did not come under the same scrutiny as women and were presumably not expected to become dependent on the state as single or even young, immature, and insufficiently educated fathers.

Similar to the young Nova Scotia woman quoted above – who seemed to shrug off responsibility for parenthood with the mere recognition that she was still just a kid, and thus not yet capable of being a responsible parent – the concerns regarding teenage sexuality relied on age-old ideas of paternalistic control over fertility: teenagers were not considered capable of responsible parenting, and some of them even agreed. Middle-class, married women, ideally in their late twenties and thirties or, even better, in their forties, were suitable activists for a kind of feminism that included responsible reproductive choices. Teenage girls, or young unmarried women more broadly, were not assumed to have accumulated the cultural capital required for making responsible choices. In these cases, then, a more conservative – or, at least, paternalistic – set of ideas prevailed: on the one hand, recoiling at the idea of discussing birth control and abortion in the classroom, but on the other, opening the doors to improved access to abortion for teens in the clinic on the supposition that single, young mothers were unfit for responsible parenthood. Moreover, many believed it was parents who represented the chief obstacle to their teen daughters, leading FPA organizers to appeal directly to teens, whether mediated through schools or directly through a comic, and to lobby governments to change the age restrictions and thereby further improve autonomous and even confidential access.

CONCLUSION

The economics of abortion and family planning had not significantly shed the fiscal logic of eugenics planners, who held that sexual sterilizations were much cheaper than supporting life in an institution. The welfare state had brought about several changes in the way that government funds supported Canadian families. The language of choice or autonomy assumed a version of life in the community, not one in an institution. Yet, the economics of family planning and support remained central to the debates over who should access abortion services and who should raise children to become good taxpaying citizens.

The discussions on abortion in the 1970s that featured in mainstream newspapers, and that appear in the documents of government and not-for-profit organizations, overwhelmingly discussed teenage pregnancy in terms of white, and presumably middle-class, adolescents. Rarely do the historical actors in these cases explicitly engage in some of the potentially more complex discussions about race, colonialism, or segregation (particularly in African Canadian communities in Nova Scotia). Inuit, First Nations, and Métis women, including teenagers, seem absent from the conversation, both as participants and as subjects. The statistics reference northern healthcare services, but rarely did the high rates of teen pregnancy in the North guide discussions about differential access or about the value of children to communities.

In contrast to discussions of people with disabilities, or of family planning within marriage, those of teenage fertility were clearly gendered. Men – whether partners, lovers, abusers, or otherwise – were seldom discussed in terms of the looming "crisis" of teenage pregnancy. Sexuality remained somewhat more opaque, mysterious, and certainly risky for teen girls. Information on sexual health had improved during the decade, but access to corresponding services, sympathetic staff, or understanding parents varied. For pregnant teens, the time-sensitive nature of pregnancy meant that they did not often have the luxury of waiting to secure the support they desired but instead had to resort to the support that was available. Confessing one's pregnancy to teachers, parents, and ultimately a TAC was proof of one's sexual activity at a moment of shifting generational perceptions of appropriate conduct.

These omissions or blind spots further underscore how the international language of population control fit awkwardly into the Canadian context. The efforts made by family planners quickly shed the veneer of global feminism, or neo-Malthusian interventions, as teenagers represented a specific, local, and economic threat to national economic stability.

Conclusion

In 2018, newly elected Ontario premier Doug Ford introduced legislation that, some commentators suggested, turned back the clock on sex education. Assuming a return to paternalism, Ford reverted to a 1990s curriculum. The *Toronto Star* characterized the changes as a "father knows best" strategy, invoking the 1950s primetime television show that depicted the growing pains of a middle-class, white American family. The *Star* columnist explained that Ford's new policy contained "no mention of consent, forcing students to read body language instead. As for (naughty) body parts, they are out again – vulvas have vanished from the vocabulary of the classroom in the early grades by order of the Progressive Conservative government (despite pleas from police and child protection authorities to equip kids with the right words in case of abuse)."[1] Students, teachers, and parents, in particular, have protested this move, arguing that sex education is critical, not just for the safety of students but also to the maintenance of civil liberties.

The language of contraception, sex education, and even population control continues to invoke political responses. Such responses are often steeped in notions of morality, but as the cases in this book demonstrate, the moral terrain is also profoundly shaped by economics. The moral ground has shifted over the course of the twentieth century, suggesting that despite the rhetoric of the 1960s sexual revolution, or the language of female liberation, concern over who controls what bodies remains open to moral interpretation.

At the end of the 1960s the concept of the population bomb captured the imagination of people and governments around the globe who, for very different reasons, became motivated to invest in deep cultural change. Women and birth control were integral components in this campaign to alter economies, environments, and social relations. There were compelling reasons to believe that the world's population was indeed exploding and to let this motivate campaigns aimed at restructuring long-standing inequities. Yet this rhetoric also revealed deeply held contradictions. Indian scholars, activists, and sisters Mira Shiva and Vandana Shiva reject population control as an "overly simplistic" notion that assumes "sustainability for the planet can only be achieved by drastic population control policies including violent and coercive contraceptive technologies for women and denial of basic health care to children." They continue: "From the women's perspective, there are two reasons why these prescriptions need to be challenged. First, it is not at all evident that population growth is the primary cause for environmental destruction. Second, coercive and hazardous population control policies work against women's health and their fundamental right to informed decision-making, and are still not effective in controlling population growth." For these reasons, Shiva and Shiva urge feminists around the globe to reconcile their relationship with birth control in a manner that takes into account the effects that these policies have on other women. Moreover, they explain that existing and persistent structures of inequality do not allow for birth control to effectively address patriarchy on a global scale. They state, "It has been noted that high birth rates are not the cause of present impoverishment; they are the response of an impoverished peasantry. When people lose all other kinds of security, children are the only economic security."[2]

When it comes to environmental degradation and energy abuse, the Global North uses 250 times as much energy as the South but has historically been slower to adopt population-control measures.[3] As Shiva and Shiva explain, "A number of people see population control policies as racist, sexist, and imperialist … [I]f stringent population policy was truly an anti-poverty measure, why have those countries in Latin American [sic] where 80 percent of the women have been sterilized become poorer and more deprived than before?"[4]

In Canada, the most aggressive application of population control targeted Indigenous women. Policy makers made very explicit connections to India as they began sanctioning physicians and public health workers to distribute birth control measures and as they removed women from their communities and families to hospitals hundreds of kilometres away to give birth and be sterilized. Allegedly responding to a global crisis in escalating birthrates, the Canadian government took its place on the international stage by justifying its actions as bringing modernity and liberty to colonized peoples within its own borders. Between 1996 and 2006 the non-Indigenous population growth rate in Canada was pegged at 8 per cent; the Indigenous growth rate was 45 per cent, suggesting that federal efforts to reduce the Indigenous birthrate have failed or even backfired.[5] According to 2018 projections, the Indigenous population is among the fastest growing in some provinces, such as Saskatchewan.[6] It seems that listening to Indigenous feminists is long overdue as we attempt to reconcile the relationships between choice, family planning, and global security.

In the 1970s, family planning and birth control captured the imagination of reformers around the world, and across the political spectrum, as fertile ground for solving problems about resource distribution and the limits of the earth's carrying capacity. The resulting liberalization of regulations around contraception also ushered in a new era of ostensibly liberated feminism, shifting the context of choice as it related to women's social capital in the ongoing discussions about fertility, global security, and population control. Not everyone had access to the same choices, and not everyone claimed responsibility for the burden of the population bomb. The international awakening of population control – or the neo-Malthusian concerns about food distribution, coupled with acute population stresses in particular areas around the globe – furnished reformers with strong economic language in the 1970s to help justify aggressive interventions.

The international discourse may have helped to galvanize support for amendments to Canada's Criminal Code, but these changes were nearly a century in the making. Canadian feminists had long lobbied for better access to reproductive health services, including maternal and infant care and, at times, abortion and contraceptive care. It is tempting to cast the amendments as triumphs of a long battle to bring women's health issues into harmony with men's health, but when it comes to reproductive health the gender dynamics are not so straightforward. Men continued to be disproportionately tasked with making the decisions, whether at the policy table, on therapeutic abortion committees, or in pulpits, while their bodies and reproductive responsibilities were largely left to their own prerogative. Some might even say that men struggled to be considered as reproductive objects as they came to define their own relationships with fertility.

Women were more often placed outside of this decision-making, bearing responsibility for pregnancy but seldom wielding the opportunity to enact changes in policy or procedure. For some women this was just more of the same. For a century at least, Indigenous women rarely had complete control over their own decisions about starting a family or keeping their children. Teenagers, as statistics indicate clearly, have a longer tradition of putting children up for adoption than of keeping and raising children as teen mothers. And for men, the context of family planning changed during the mid-twentieth century, from a perception that "father knows best" to the notion that fathers are responsible too.

After 1969, contraception quickly shifted from being something that was considered taboo in public conversation, and perhaps even proof of sexual promiscuity, to a badge of responsibility – at least, for some. Heterosexual teens in the 1970s seemed caught between exercising their newfound sexual freedom to engage in premarital intercourse, and admitting that they were doing it. Promiscuity still cast a dark shadow on sex as evidence of immorality or irresponsibility that signalled challenges ahead for establishing a healthy, financially secure, nuclear family. While public health officials and family planners may have argued otherwise, the spectre of morality continued to hover over the use of contraception, making it difficult to liberalize sex without also deregulating access to birth control.

The expansion of welfare-state services, including substantial spending and service provision in health under Medicare, created among citizens a different relationship with the state and different expectations when it came to family planning options. Women were increasingly expected to get an education before getting married, and presumably before having children. People who had lived in custodial care facilities because of physical, mental, or intellectual disabilities were increasingly part of the single-family dwelling, consequently changing the contours of care and altering family dynamics when it came to providing home-care services. At the same time, caring for unexpected grandchildren or dependent adult children also created strains on household income and demands on family members, who might otherwise be income earners, to stay at home to engage in the (unpaid) care economy.

Contrary to claims that the welfare state provided greater supports for Canadian families, it also coincided with the deregulation of some forms of state support, namely long-stay institutions. While this was a positive move, given what we have learned about the experiences of those who were institutionalized, it effectively shifted the onus of care onto families at precisely the moment when family planning and family values assumed new meanings. The responsible choice was not necessarily clear when reproduction might have meant reducing the number of income earners in the household, or when keeping a child meant giving up an education. These kinds of scenarios played out across different bodies but cut across geographical lines with remarkable consistency.

Every region in Canada registered concerns with the idea that teens were seemingly engaging in unprotected sex, thereby exposing themselves to infections as well as unwanted pregnancies, both of which allegedly had the potential to cause long-term problems for young people. A nationwide lack of consistent service provision also placed people across a range of categories of race, ability, and gender in precarious positions in which they took matters into their own hands, namely by travelling to a jurisdiction that provided the necessary services. Many women living in the Northwest Territories, for example, travelled south, away from their families, to procure hospital-based services. Not all of these women took this path willingly, but their need to obtain services underscores the uneven distribution of health care that underpinned these decisions to travel. Similarly, women seeking abortions that were not available in their home regions travelled, if they had the means, to nearby jurisdictions to secure the desired surgery. For women in Saskatchewan or Manitoba this often meant going to Alberta, or leaving the country. For parents of disabled children in Ontario, this meant seeking out-of-province services to have their children sterilized after the province had placed a moratorium on sterilizations of dependent adults in 1978. The persistence of individuals suggests that despite the various barriers that frustrated their access to these services, family planning at the individual level continued to defy both laws and moral arguments against them.

One of the biggest challenges we faced in writing this book was trying to uncover an underlying logic to family planning strategies in this period, especially when it came to marginalized populations. Just when we felt confident that we had sorted out the motivations and methods applied to one group of Canadians, we turned to another case study and the ground shifted. Our conclusion, then, is rather unsatisfying in terms of crafting an overall argument about the nature of family planning in Canada. Bringing the analysis down to the level of individuals readily reveals that these decisions were frequently messy and often involved outside factors, such as morals and economics, as much as concerns about health, or access to services, or fears about the impact of pregnancy on one's future as a parent, employee, or citizen. Often the high-level discussions did not match the tenor of those conversations at the individual level, but the results were such that families shopped for the responses they needed at the time they needed them or made do with the outcomes regardless of the laws.

We ultimately conclude that the relationship between population control and birth control has a long history – one that continued into the 1970s in ways that were more consistent with than different from the past. While some of the rhetoric shifted, the power dynamics remained in place and, at least during that decade, the traditional lines of authority over reproductive bodies remained intact. Canada's healthcare policy arena created specific conditions for the introduction of new reproductive technologies.[7] Medicare ensured that tubal ligations were within reach for women seeking sterilization surgeries who did not necessarily consider the personal financial cost, but who also did not rely on vasectomized men to manage the birth control decisions in a family. Birth control in the 1970s retained trappings of earlier eugenics debates but also generated new perspectives or a "newgenic" approach to controlling reproduction and sexuality among people considered disabled, genetically undesirable, or incapable of taking care of their own menstrual hygiene. Some of those discussions did not deviate from a paternalistic approach to determining the reproductive fate of women and men considered irresponsible on account of their disability, despite legal changes that ensured they remained in a different category of ability and choice.

As Canadians in the twenty-first century face the prospect of greater environmental change, with increased numbers of forest fires, heat waves, and ice storms, devastating hurricanes and prolonged droughts, the environmental cry for population control may again be getting louder. Population control remains a significant theme in the global economy, as rising levels of wealth create even greater levels of consumption. Fertility seems to be taking a back seat in these discussions, in the latest iteration of a Malthusian turn. Countries that had introduced drastic measures to control fertility have started relaxing those same policies while consuming even more. China's one-child policy has been relaxed, while the country has pledged to wean itself off of coal as its main energy source.[8] Africa now claims to be home to the countries with the highest birthrates, many of which also coincide with the lowest life expectancies.[9] During the 1970s, Canadian decision-makers looked to international crises to help inform local decisions about controlling reproduction in an effort to reduce the stress on the environment and populations. It remains to be seen whether Canadians will continue to look beyond our borders to craft sustainable solutions in a manner that balances human rights with environmental needs. Moreover, as 1970s thinkers looked to the Global South for proof of population density, twenty-first-century critics are beginning to turn the lens toward consumption as one of the main culprits of environmental calamity. Perhaps in Canada, one of the biggest consumers on the planet, it is time to look for local solutions to global problems. We may need to reframe population control by embracing, rather than eschewing, the relationship between environmental destruction and population growth. We may need to figure out how to control our consumption before we consider recommending that others control their fertility.

Notes

INTRODUCTION

1 Huxley, *Brave New World* (1932), 7.
2 Huxley, *Brave New World Revisited* (1958), 26.
3 See Tone, *Devices and Desires* (2001).
4 See, especially, Lombardo, *Three Generations* (2008); Stern, *Eugenic Nation* (2016); Kline, *Building a Better Race* (2001); and Stepan, *Hour of Eugenics* (1996).
5 Ehrlich, *Population Bomb* (1968).
6 According to the World Data Atlas, in 1968 India had a population of 531,513,824 and China had a population of 774,510,000. "India: Total Population," World Data Atlas, n.d., accessed 18 February 2020, https://knoema.com/atlas/India/Population; "China: Total Population," World Data Atlas, n.d., accessed 18 February 2020, https://knoema.com/atlas/China/topics/Demographics/Population/Population.
7 Connelly, *Fatal Misconception* (2008), ix.
8 Wikipedia, s.v. "Paul R. Ehrlich," accessed 13 December 2019, https://en.wikipedia.org/wiki/Paul_R._Ehrlich.
9 Wolfers and Wolfers, "Vasectomania" (1973), 198.
10 For more on this topic, see Dyck, "Abortion and Birth Control" (2017); and Marsh and Ronner, *Fertility Doctor* (2008).
11 We elaborate on this point in chapter 1, where the sole female member of Parliament points out that Canada cannot distribute birth control to other countries while ignoring the demands from women for access to contraception within its own borders. Canada, Parliament, House of Commons, *Debates*, 28th Parl., 1st sess., 8 (14 May 1969): 8708.

12 "The Population Bomb, 50 Years Later: A Conversation with Paul Ehrlich," Climate One, n.d., accessed 7 May 2018, https://climateone.org/audio/population-bomb-50-years-later-conversation-paul-ehrlich.

13 For more on this topic, see Blake, *From Rights to Needs* (2009).

14 For a more in-depth study of the impact of the Pill on married women in Canada, see Haynes, "Great Emancipator" (2012).

15 For example, see Kevles, *In the Name of Eugenics* (1995).

16 Bulmer, *Francis Galton* (2003), 32.

17 Mazumdar, *Eugenics, Human Genetics* (1992); Dorr, *Segregation's Science* (2008); Paul, *Politics of Heredity* (1998); Pichot, *Pure Society* (2009); Lombardo, *Three Generations*.

18 McLaren and McLaren, *Bedroom and the State* (1986).

19 Pichot, *Pure Society*; Kevles, *In the Name of Eugenics*; Weindling, *Victims and Survivors* (2014).

20 Backhouse, *Prejudice and Petticoats* (1991); Sethna and Hewitt, *Just Watch Us* (2018); Sethna and Davis, eds., *Abortion across Borders* (2019); Appleby, *Responsible Parenthood* (1999); McTavish, "Abortion in New Brunswick" (2015); Stettner, ed., *Without Apology* (2016); Baillargeon, *Babies for the Nation* (2009); Stote, *Act of Genocide* (2015); Hansen and King, *Sterilized by the State* (2013).

21 Dunphy, *Morgentaler* (2003); Stettner, Burnett, and Hay, eds., *Abortion* (2017).

22 Dowbiggin, *Sterilization Movement* (2008); Connelly, *Fatal Misconception*; Bashford, *Global Population* (2014).

23 Murphy, *Economization of Life* (2017), 46.

24 Margaret Sanger made this case in her own campaign. See Katz, Engelman, and Hajo, eds., *Selected Papers of Margaret Sanger* (2016).

25 McLaren, *Our Own Master Race* (1990); Dyck, *Facing Eugenics* (2013).

26 McLaren and McLaren, *Bedroom and the State*, 12.

27 Watkins, *On the Pill* (1998), 11.

28 Section 179 of the 1892 Canadian Criminal Code, quoted in McLaren and McLaren, *Bedroom and the State*, 19.

29 Molyneaux, "Controlling Conception" (2011), 68–9.

30 Marsh and Ronner, *Fertility Doctor*.

31 Canada, Parliament, House of Commons, *Debates*, 14 May 1969, 8708.

32 Canada, Department of National Health and Welfare, *Current Status of Family Planning in Canada* (Ottawa, September 1971), 8, RG29 (records of Department of National Health and Welfare), acc. 1995-96/212, vol. 3, file 4440-2-22, part 1, Library and Archives Canada (hereafter LAC).

33 Throughout our analysis we rely on Foucauldian ideas, especially those elaborated upon in Foucault, *Discipline and Punish* (1977) and *Madness and Civilization* (2001) and his concept of governmentality, linked to ideas of biopower, articulated especially in *Birth of Biopolitics* (2008).

34 Some of the scholarship focusing on the 1960s in Canada reinforces the idea that this period ruptured Canadian identity along a variety of lines – for example, in changing relations with Indigenous people, acknowledging student protests across the nation, or confronting the political realities of the Front de libération du Québec – altering the way that Canadians thought of themselves as a nation and as citizens. See, for example, Palmer, *Canada's 1960s* (2009); Owram, *Born at the Right Time* (1996); and Igartua, *Other Quiet Revolution* (2011).

35 See Campbell, Clément, and Kealey, eds., *Debating Dissent* (2012).

36 Several interviews presented in a 2003 PBS documentary express this sentiment; see *The Pill*, produced, directed, and written by Chana Gazit, aired 24 February 2003, https://www.pbs.org/wgbh/americanexperience/films/pill/.

37 Leon, *Image of God* (2013).

38 See Stevenson, *Intimate Integration* (2020).

39 Ing, "Canada's Indian Residential Schools" (2006).

40 Stevenson, "Intimate Integration" (2015).

41 See Desjardins, "La construction anthropologique" (2001).

42 Ladd-Taylor, "Contraception or Eugenics?" (2014).

43 Dyck, *Facing Eugenics*, 137–42; Watkins, *On the Pill*; Lord, *Condom Nation* (2010); Parry, *Broadcasting Birth Control* (2013).

44 Shropshire, "What's a Guy to Do?" (2014); Fleming and Joyce, "Elective Sterilization" (1968).

45 Dodds, *Voluntary Male Sterilization* (1970).

46 See Williams with Gill, "Campus Campaigns" ([2014]).

CHAPTER ONE

1 Quoted in McLaren and McLaren, *Bedroom and the State*, 9.

2 Canada, Parliament, House of Commons, *Debates*, 28th Parl., 1st sess., 7 (17 April 1969): 7630, 7631.

3 Deighton, "Nature of Eugenic Thought" (2018); Dyck, "Eugenics in Canada" (2018). For a more robust survey of eugenics around the world, see Bashford and Levine, eds., *Oxford Handbook* (2010).

4 Dyck, *Facing Eugenics*; Ladd-Taylor, *Fixing the Poor* (2017); Malacrida, *Special Hell* (2015); Samson, "Eugenics in the Community" (2014), 146–7.

5 Dyck, "Sterilization and Birth Control" (2014), 178–82.

6 American women of color whose communities experienced reproductive
   oppression developed the notion of reproductive justice in the early 1990s.
   As an intersectional theory it recognizes that a woman's ability to control
   her reproduction is linked to the socioeconomic conditions in her community – her race and class – and not just a matter of individual choice and
   access. Ross, "What Is Reproductive Justice?" (2019); see also Gurr,
   Reproductive Justice (2015), 32.

7 Bock, "Racism and Sexism" (1983); Briggs, "Discourses of 'Forced
   Sterilization'" (1998), 34; see also Harris, ed., *Schism of '68* (2016).

8 Feldberg, "On the Cutting Edge" (2003), 129; Leavitt, *Brought to Bed*
   (1993).

9 Molyneaux, "Controlling Conception," 66.

10 "Spreading the Word about the Pill," *Toronto Star*, 10 April 1967, 1.

11 On this topic, see, for example, O'Brien, *Framing the Moron* (2013);
   Ladd-Taylor, *Fixing the Poor*; Dyck, *Facing Eugenics*; and Lombardo,
   Three Generations.

12 See, especially, Ladd-Taylor, *Fixing the Poor*.

13 "Abortion Law Reform Said Partial Answer," *Leader Post* (Regina),
   26 October 1967, 19.

14 Royal Commission on the Status of Women, *Report*, Ottawa, 7 December
   1979, 286.

15 Christine Chisholm argues that Canada was unique in not recommending
   a "eugenics clause" or another clause in the amendment to allow for
   abortion in the case of confirmed disability or malformation of the child.
   Despite this outcome, newspaper reports at the time confirm that these
   issues were being raised by advocates of abortion reform. See Chisholm,
   "Curious Case of Thalidomide" (2016).

16 "Abortion Law Reform," *Leader Post*.

17 Ibid.

18 "Legalized Abortion," *Star Phoenix* (Saskatoon), 5 August 1967, 21.

19 Hardin, "1960" (1964).

20 See Orr, *Panic Diaries* (2006); Roszak, *Making of a Counter Culture*
   (1969).

21 Blake, *From Rights to Needs* (2009), 179.

22 Ibid., 185.

23 Canada, Parliament, House of Commons, *Debates*, 28th Parl., 1st sess.,
   7 (18 April 1969): 7691, 7704.

24 For a counterpoint, see Lišková, *Sexual Liberation, Socialist Style* (2018).

25 Canada, Parliament, House of Commons, *Debates*, 18 April 1969, 7704.

26 Canada, Parliament, House of Commons, *Debates*, 28th Parl., 1st sess., 8 (28 April 1969): 8079.

27 Canada, Parliament, House of Commons, *Debates*, 28th Parl., 1st sess., 8 (13 May 1969): 8632.

28 Canada, Parliament, House of Commons, *Debates*, 28th Parl., 1st sess., 8 (1 May 1969): 8633.

29 Canada, Parliament, House of Commons, *Debates*, 28 April 1969: 8079.

30 Canada, Parliament, House of Commons, *Debates*, 18 April 1969: 7638.

31 Canada, Parliament, House of Commons, *Debates*, 17 April 1969: 7639.

32 Rosenfeld, *Orgiastic Near East* (1968), 7.

33 Canada, Parliament, House of Commons, *Debates*, 17 April 1969: 7638.

34 Canada, Parliament, House of Commons, *Debates*, 28th Parl., 1st sess., 8 (5 May 1969): 8314.

35 Canada, Parliament, House of Commons, *Debates*, 13 May 1969: 8635.

36 Palmer, "Lonely, Tragic" (2011), 638.

37 Egan and Gardner, "Reproductive Freedom" (2016), 131.

38 Palmer, "Abortion on Trial" (2017), 115.

39 Canada, Parliament, House of Commons, *Debates*, 28th Parl., 1st sess., 7 (25 April 1969): 7966

40 *Bill C-150: Criminal Law Amendment Act*, 1968–69, SC 1968–69, c 38.

41 S. d'Estrube, letter to the editor, *Peninsula Times*, 29 April 1970, B4.

42 For an in-depth study, see Sethna and Hewitt, "Clandestine Operations" (2009).

43 Canada, Parliament, House of Commons, *Debates*, 28th Parl., 3rd sess., 1 (8 May 1970): 6741.

44 Quoted from the Royal Commission for the Status of Women, homepage: https://cfc-swc.gc.ca/abu-ans/wwad-cqnf/roycom/index-en.html, accessed April 19, 2020.

45 Royal Commission on the Status of Women, *Report*, 5.

46 Ibid., 7, translated from Lilar, *Le malentendu* (1969), 234.

47 Royal Commission on the Status of Women, *Report*, 10–11.

48 Ibid., 17.

49 Ibid., 229.

50 Ibid.

51 The report's section on family makes this point clearly; see, especially, ibid., 229–33.

52 Ibid., 238.

53 Ibid., 275.

54 Ibid.

55 Ibid.

56 Ibid., 278.
57 Ibid., 279–80.
58 Ibid., 281.
59 Ibid., 282.
60 Ibid., 284.
61 Ibid., 285.
62 Ibid.

CHAPTER TWO

1 Marc Lalonde to Laurent Picard, 6 April 1973, RG 29, vol. 2870, file 851-1-5 pt. 3a, LAC.
2 Cardinal, *Unjust Society* (1969), 1.
3 Sethna et al., "Choice, Interrupted" (2013), 31.
4 The government's position is articulated most clearly in the records of the Indian Health Service, an agency within the Department of Health and Welfare. Moreover, until 1988 the federal government was directly responsible for the health care of all Territorial residents, including Indigenous people; the federal minister of health was the health minister for the Territories.
5 Boyer, "First Nations, Métis and Inuit Health" (2011), 184.
6 Primeau, "Social History" (1998).
7 Stote, "Act of Genocide" (2012), 2.
8 Since published as Stote, *Act of Genocide.*
9 A.D. Hunt to M.L. Webb, 1 June 1973, RG 29, vol.. 2870, file 851-1-5, pt. 3B, LAC.
10 Letter to the Department of National Health and Welfare from Public Health Committee [translated from Inuktitut syllabics; signed by 5 women, names and location withheld], 19 December 1976, RG 29, vol. 2870, file 851-1-5, pt. 4, LAC.
11 Briggs, "Discourses of 'Forced Sterilization'" (1998), 34.
12 Ibid., 30.
13 The Report of the Royal Commission on the Status of Women in Canada, filed in 1970, included recommendations to end sex discrimination in the Indian Act. See Green, "Taking Account" (2007), 24. The two primary groups that formed at this time were Indian Rights for Indian Women (1970) and the Native Women's Association of Canada (1974).
14 The three significant lawsuits were *Attorney General of Canada v. Lavell* (1973), *Bédard v. Isaac et al.* (1972), and *Sandra Lovelace v. Canada*

(1981). The Indian Act was amended in 1985 by Bill C-31, which
reinstated some of the disenfranchised.

15 Cardinal, *Unjust Society*, 140.

16 Barker, "Gender, Sovereignty," 137.

17 Green, "Taking Account," 20; St. Denis, "Feminism Is for Everybody"
(2007), 33. See also Snyder, "Indigenous Feminist Legal Theory"
(2014), 381.

18 Osennontion (Kane) and Skonaganleh:rá, "Our World" (1989), 15.

19 Turpel, "Patriarchy and Paternalism" (1993), 191, 180.

20 Ouellette, *Fourth World* (2002), 85. Ouellette conducted her research in
the 1980s building explicitly on Manuel and Posluns, *Fourth World* (1974).

21 Ouellette, *Fourth World*, 84; see also Turpel, "Patriarchy and Paternalism,"
180–1.

22 Udel, "Revision and Resistance" (2001), 45.

23 A US federal investigation in 1976 uncovered the gritty details of sterilizations of over three thousand women between the ages of fifteen and forty-
four that ignored or violated safeguards intended to ensure informed
consent and to prevent coercion. Many of these girls and women were in
fact teenagers who were sterilized under the auspices of appendectomies,
without their knowledge or consent. Udel, "Revision and Resistance," 46;
see also Lawrence, "Indian Health Service" (2000).

24 Udel, "Revision and Resistance," 45–6.

25 Luther, "Whose 'Distinctive Culture'?" (2010).

26 Green, "Taking Account," 23, 24.

27 Ibid., 18.

28 Suzack, "Indigenous Feminisms" (2015), 262.

29 *Pauktuutit Inuit Women's Association*, "Pauktuutit" (1989).

30 Kaufert and O'Neil, "Cooptation and Control" (1990), 439.

31 McCallum, "Last Frontier" (2005).

32 For the sake of consistency, we will use Indian Health Service (IHS)
to refer to the bureaucracy responsible for health care. Known as Indian
Health Service when it was housed in the Department of Indian Affairs,
it retained the name when health services were transferred to National
Health and Welfare in 1945. Reflecting an increasing responsibility in the
North, the name was changed to the Indian and Northern Health Service
(INHS) in 1955. In 1962 another government reorganization saw the elim-
ination of INHS and the creation of the Medical Services Branch (MSB),
an amalgamation of seven former independent services: Civil Aviation,
Civil Service Health, Northern Health, Quarantine, Immigration, Sick

Mariners, and the largest, Indian Health Service. In 2000 it was renamed the First Nations and Inuit Health Branch (FNIHB).

33 *An Act Respecting Sexual Sterilization*, S.B.C. 1933, c 59.

34 Indian hospitals, racially segregated institutions, were established by the federal government in the 1930s and 1940s to treat First Nations and Inuit patients while isolating them from community hospitals. See Lux, *Separate Beds* (2016).

35 Among other local Indigenous dignitaries, Henry Kelly, councillor for the Tsimshian at Port Simpson (Lax Kw'alaams), attended the opening ceremony and spoke of the hospital as a "milestone along the road of progress in the new deal promised by the government of Canada for my people." Quoted in "Formal Opening of Finely-Equipped Hospital at Miller Bay for TB Cases," *Evening Empire* (Prince Rupert), 17 September 1946.

36 Coates, *Best Left as Indians* (1991), 102.

37 G.R. Howell to W.S. Barclay, 9 August 1954, RG29, vol. 2869, file 851-1-5, pt. 1, LAC.

38 Eric Preston, "Observations – Miller Bay Indian Hospital," 6 June 1956, RG29, vol. 2598, file 800-1-D579, pt. 1, LAC.

39 P. Moore to R.E. Curran, chief, legal division, 5 October 1954, RG29, vol. 2869, file 851-1-5, pt. 1, LAC.

40 Eugenics Board, minutes (Binder 1), 31 May 1937, n.p., University of Alberta. See also T.R.L. MacInnes to director of Indian Affairs Branch, Department of Mines and Resources, 11 May 1937; and G.C. Laight, Indian agent, Edmonton, to director of Indian Affairs Branch, Department of Mines and Resources, 11 May 1937, re: Sterilization of Indian Cases, both at University of Alberta.

41 Dyck, *Facing Eugenics*, 12.

42 Medical superintendent to Indian agent, Department of Indian Affairs, Edmonton, 26 May 1937, in Eugenics Board, minutes (Binder 1), 31 May 1937, University of Alberta.

43 Dyck, *Facing Eugenics*, 3.

44 "Form 7819: Application for Medical Treatment," RG29, vol. 2869, file 851-1-5, pt. 1, LAC.

45 J.C. Hanson, department solicitor, to Office of Provincial Secretary, Government of BC, 8 October 1954, RG29, vol. 2869, file 851-1-5 pt. 1, LAC.

46 Moore to W.S. Barclay, 8 December 1954, RG29, vol. 2869, file 851-1-5, pt. 1, LAC.

47 O'Neil, "Self-Determination" (1988), 36.

48 Kaufert and O'Neil, "Cooptation and Control," 438–9.

49 "Supply of Contraceptives," handwritten memo, 24 [or 29] December 1955, RG29, vol. 2869, file 851-1-5, pt. 1, LAC.

50 Until the 1969 amendments, the Criminal Code stated that "every one commits an offence who knowingly, without lawful justification or excuse … (c) offers to sell, advertises, publishes an advertisement of, or has for sale or disposal any means, instructions, medicine, drug, or article intended or represented as a method of preventing conception or causing abortion or miscarriage." Cited in Appleby, *Responsible Parenthood*, 3. Appleby notes that a defence to the charge could be found in proving the claim that the actions served the public good.

51 "Legal Aspects of Sterilization" (1949): 53.

52 McLaren and McLaren, *Bedroom and the State*, 123.

53 Dr D. Blake, "Policy re Supply of Contraceptive Materials," memo to file, 3 January 1956, RG29, vol. 2869, file 851-1-5, pt. 1, LAC.

54 The IHS "Application for Medical Treatment" form explicitly states that "no one except the Director may approve elective surgery, treatment for cosmetic purposes only, or the use of expensive materials." RG29, vol. 2869, file 851-1-5 pt. 1, LAC.

55 Appleby, *Responsible Parenthood*, 6.

56 W.L. Falconer to all Zones in Foothills Region "Drugs – Contraceptives", 7 August 1962, RG29, vol. 2869, file 851-1-5, pt. 1, LAC.

57 Thalidomide, a sedative, first appeared in West Germany in 1957; the connection between thalidomide and severe birth defects convinced the German developers to recall the drug in November 1961. In Canada the Food and Drug Directorate had approved thalidomide for sale in April 1961; it was not taken off the market until February 1962. Clow, "Illness of Nine Months' Duration" (2003).

58 Ortho Pharmaceutical (Canada) Ltd., "Important – Drug Caution Ortho-Novum Tablets," 9 August 1962; P.E. Moore to all regional superintendents, "Enovid," 10 September 1962, both in RG29, vol. 2869, file 851-1-5 pt. 1, LAC.

59 Moore, "How Do These Prices Compare with Enovid?," memo, 6 September 1962, RG29, vol. 2869, file 851-1-5, pt. 1, LAC.

60 Moore to all regional superintendents, "Enovid," LAC. Other side effects included nausea, gastrointestinal disturbances, breast tenderness, weight gain, and breakthrough bleeding. In the United States, by August 1962, there were twenty-eight reported cases of death and disease from blood clots linked to Enovid, the only brand on the American market at the time; although acknowledged by physicians, the Pill's dangerous side effects

were not widely understood by the public until after 1969. Watkins, *On the Pill*, 81, 103.

61 M.E. Gordon, assistant Pacific zone superintendent, to zone superintendent, Miller Bay Indian Hospital, 24 September 1965, RG29, vol. 2869, file 851-1-5, pt. 1a, LAC.

62 Some remained suspicious of the government's motives and methods. In 1974 a man from Toronto posed an unanswerable question to the government: "Are you still permitting the pill being passed off as a vitamin pill to the Indians, Metis and Inuits [*sic*]?" 14 December 1974, RG29, vol. 2870, file 851-1-5, pt. 3b, LAC.

63 A.R. Kaufman, Kitchener, ON, to P.E. Moore, 28 November 1963; Moore to Kaufman, 6 December 1963, both in RG29, vol. 2869, file 851-1-5 pt. 1, LAC.

64 Briggs, *Reproducing Empire* (2002), 116.

65 The Population Council, using Rockefeller and Ford Foundation funds, promoted contraceptive research centres and supplied national programs with technology and expertise. By 1968, 90 per cent of IPPF funds originated in the United States. Connelly, "Seeing beyond the State" (2006), 221–2, 226.

66 Ibid., 202.

67 McLaren and McLaren, *Bedroom and the State*, 134.

68 Appleby, *Responsible Parenthood*, 47.

69 Blacker, "International Planned Parenthood Federation" (1964).

70 Connelly, "Seeing beyond the State," 220.

71 Cited in Appleby, *Responsible Parenthood*, 45.

72 H.A. Proctor to all regional superintendents, 27 August 1965, "Birth Control," RG29, vol. 2869, file 851-1-5, pt.1, LAC. Percy Moore retired in July 1965, after twenty years as director, and was replaced by his long-serving assistant, H.A. Proctor.

73 J.D. Galbraith to regional superintendent, 8 September 1965, RG29, vol. 2869, file 851-1-5, pt. 1, LAC.

74 M.L. Webb to director general, 13 September 1965, RG29, vol. 2869, file 851-1-5, pt. 1, LAC.

75 G.D. Gray to zone superintendent, 3 September 1965, RG29, vol. 2869, file 851-1-5, pt. 1, LAC.

76 S. Mallick to director, 15 December 1964, RG29, vol. 2869, file 851-1-5, pt. 1, LAC.

77 S. Mallick to regional superintendent, 8 September 1965, RG29, vol. 2869, file 851-1-5, pt. 1, LAC.

78 Rebecca Kluchin argues that neo-eugenics in the post–World War II
period, like eugenics before it, rested on definitions of reproductive fitness.
For neo-eugenicists, certain "defects" (such as poverty, illegitimacy, and
criminality) were reproduced, but culture, rather than genes, was the
means of transmission. Kluchin, *Fit to be Tied* (2011), 3.

79 T.J. Orford to director, 3 September 1965, RG29, vol. 2869, file 851-1-5,
pt.1, LAC.

80 M.P.D. Waldron to director, 2 September 1965, RG29, vol. 2869,
file 851-1-5, pt.1, LAC.

81 R.D. Thompson to director general, 13 September 1965, RG29, vol. 2869,
file 851-1-5, pt.1, LAC.

82 Zone superintendent, Inuvik, to regional superintendent, 8 September 1965,
RG29, vol. 2869, file 851-1-5, pt. 1, LAC.

83 R.A. Sprenger to regional superintendent, 7 September 1965, RG29,
vol. 2869, file 851-1-5, pt. 1, LAC.

84 G.C. Butler, chief medical officer, to S.M. Hodgson, commissioner, "Brief
on Birth Control," 11 June 1968, RG29, vol. 2869, file 851-1-5, pt. 1, LAC.

85 "N.W.T. Will Offer Birth Control Facts," [Edmonton] *Journal*, n.d.
[27 February 1968], RG29, vol. 2869, file 851-1-5, pt. 1, LAC. Before
1974 the governing council was composed of a mix of elected members
and Ottawa appointees.

86 K.G. Basavarajappa and Bali Ram, "Section A: Population and
Migration," *Historical Statistics of Canada*, Statistics Canada, Ottawa,
July 1999, http://www.statcan.gc.ca/pub/11-516-x/pdf/5500092-eng.pdf.

87 "Canada's Shame," [Edmonton] *Journal*, n.d. [28 February 1968], RG29,
vol. 2869, file 851-1-5, pt. 1, LAC.

88 According to Trudeau, "The Just Society will be one in which our Indian
and Inuit population will be encouraged to assume the full rights of citizenship through policies which will give them both greater responsibility
for their own future and more meaningful equality of opportunity."
Trudeau, "Just Society" (1998), 16.

89 Canada, *Statement of the Government of Canada on Indian Policy* [White
Paper] (Ottawa, 1969), http://www.aadnc-aandc.gc.ca/DAM/DAM-
INTER-HQ/STAGING/texte-text/cp1969_1100100010190_eng.pdf.

90 Indeed, foreshadowing the White Paper, for much of the previous decade
IHS had been attempting to off-load its responsibilities for health care
to the provinces by restricting services and closing its Indian hospitals.
Indigenous organizations, particularly in Alberta and Saskatchewan,
were politically active in resisting government attempts to abrogate their

treaty rights. IHS regional director, "Amendments to the Medical Services
Program," memorandum, 26 February 1968, RG29, vol. 2936, file 851-1-
x400, pt. 2(b), LAC; Harold Cardinal to All Chiefs and Band Councils,
13 June 1969, RG29, vol. 2936, file 851-1-x400, pt. 3(a), LAC.

91 Along with the Alberta Chiefs' response – the "Red Paper," or *Citizens
Plus* (Indian Chiefs of Alberta, *Citizens Plus* [June 1970], http://caid.ca/
RedPaper1970.pdf) – other counterproposals to the White Paper included
the Union of British Columbia Chiefs' *A Declaration of Indian Rights*
(1970); Manitoba Indian Brotherhood's *Wahbung: Our Tomorrows*
(1971); Association of Iroquois and Allied Indians' *Position Paper* (1971).
Weaver, *Making Canadian Indian Policy* (1981), 188–9.

92 Cardinal, *Unjust Society*, 1, 126, 139; Weaver, *Making Canadian
Indian Policy.*

93 The Family Planning Division produced pamphlets targeting two groups
in particular: "Birth Control ... Facts for Teenagers" and "To Live and Be
Free," suitable for use by "lower socio-economic groups." Brian Stehler,
Family Planning Federation, to Dr Lennox, RG29, vol. 2869, file 851-1-5,
pt. 2, LAC. It also directed the Canadian International Development
Agency to provide assistance to population control programs in the
third world. Appleby, *Responsible Parenthood*, 217.

94 J.H. Wiebe to professional staff, "Confidential, Family Planning Policy,"
8 October 1971, RG29, vol. 2869, file 851-1-5, pt. 2, LAC.

95 The other principles stated that planning could not be freely undertaken
without sufficient information, education, and instruction. Ibid.

96 The memo states that the policy was developed at a February 1971 meeting with departmental officials and representatives of "national agencies
which were active in support of family planning programs" that also
included the Canadian Medical Association, the Association of Canadian
Social Workers, the Canadian Nurses Association, and the short-lived
Centre de planning familial du Québec.

97 Connelly, "Seeing beyond the State," 222.

98 M.L. Webb, assistant deputy minister, to Ian Watson, MP, 28 February
1972, RG29, vol. 2869, file 851-1-5, pt. 2, LAC.

99 Wiebe to professional staff, "Confidential, Family Planning Policy," LAC.

100 Minister to J.N. Crawford, deputy minister, 12 February 1969, RG29,
vol. 2869, file 851-1-5, pt. 1, LAC.

101 Wiebe to professional staff, "Confidential, Family Planning Policy," LAC.

102 Canada, Parliament, House of Commons *Debates*, 28th Parl., 3rd sess.,
1 (9 October 1970): 16.

103 Canada, Parliament, House of Commons *Debates*, 28th Parl., 3rd sess.,
     1 (14 October 1970): 111.
104 "Eskimo Sterilization Inhumane – Lewis," *Edmonton Journal*,
     10 October 1970.
105 G.C. Butler, regional director, to zone directors, 29 October 1970, RG29,
     vol. 2869, file 851-1-5, pt. 2 LAC.
106 Native American women were particular targets of sterilization abuse in the
     1960s and 1970s in the United States. Kluchin, *Fit to Be Tied*, 8, 108–9.
107 By the early 1980s, all women were evacuated to hospitals for childbirth.
     Kaufert and O'Neil, "Cooptation and Control," 431.
108 G.D. Gray to zone superintendent, 3 September 1965, RG29, vol. 2869,
     file 851-1-5, pt. 1, LAC. The Yellowknife Family Planning Clinic, a mem-
     ber of the FPFC, visited all postpartum patients in the Yellowknife hospi-
     tal. Director, Northern Region, to assistant deputy minister, 24 February
     1972, RG29, vol. 2869, file 851-1-5, pt. 2, LAC. The practice of health-
     care workers urging Indigenous women to undergo tubal ligation after
     giving birth continued in 2015. "Sterilization Pressure Odious," editorial,
     Star Phoenix (Saskatoon), 17 November 2015.
109 *Weekend*, aired 1 April 1973, CBC Television, transcript, RG29, vol. 2870,
     file 851-1-5, pt. 3a, LAC. "Anna" is not her real name. It is not clear
     whether the television broadcast identified all the individuals interviewed,
     though their names, communities, and personal medical histories appear
     in the archival record. For that reason, we decline to identify communities
     or individuals by name.

CHAPTER THREE

1 Anderson, *Recognition of Being* (2000), 83.
2 Smith, *Decolonizing Methodologies* (2012).
3 Anderson, *Recognition of Being*, 17; Lavell-Harvard and Corbiere Lavell,
     "Thunder Spirits" (2006), 5–6.
4 Canada, Department of National Health and Welfare, *Current Status
     of Family Planning*, 6, 17.
5 Ibid., 2.
6 Ibid., 18, 26.
7 Ibid., 10.
8 Ibid., 13.
9 The report put the national population at 21,377,000 and the Indigenous
     population at 235,964. Ibid.

10 C.A.D. Ringrose, "Birth Control – Current Methods of Contraception"
    Alberta Native Women's second annual convention, 3–6 March 1969,
    Voice of Alberta Native Women's Society, GR1979.0152, box 8, file 85,
    Provincial Archives of Alberta (PAA).

11 Ringrose, "Birth Control," PAA.

12 "Recommendations of the First National Conference on Family Planning,"
    in Schlesinger, ed., *Family Planning in Canada* (1974), 119, 121, 124.

13 "Background Notes for Discussion of Birth Control," March 1975, RG29,
    acc. 1990-91/248, vol. 10, file 0141-7-B1, LAC.

14 "Resolutions passed at the Alberta conference on family planning,
    May 16–18, 1973," RG29, vol. 1767, file 45-14-1, pt. 2, LAC.

15 Family Planning Association of BC, Newsletter, 30 June 1973, VI, RG29,
    acc. 1987-88/254, vol. 2, file 150-1-24, pt. 2, LAC.

16 Connelly, *Fatal Misconception*, 90.

17 Family Planning Association of BC, "Community Responses, Needs and
    Priorities, Interim Report," May 1973, n.p., RG29, acc. 1987-88/254, V 2,
    file 150-1-24, pt. 2, LAC.

18 Ibid.

19 Family Planning Association of Manitoba, "Constitution" and "Proposed
    Activities for 1975," n.d., MG28, I 463, Records of Planned Parenthood
    Federation of Canada, vol. 14, file 12, LAC.

20 "Directions for the Future: Needs and Priorities – A Birth Control and
    Sex Education Conference," October 1974, 64, Records of Planned
    Parenthood Ontario, F825-2, box B286910, Archives of Ontario (AO).

21 Ibid., 64–5.

22 Donald K. Herald to Hon. J. Buchanan, 19 November 1974,
    F825-MU-4407, box B285908, AO.

23 For example, Vancouver's Indigenous population, 530 in 1961, had risen
    to 16,080 by 1981; Toronto's population grew from 1,196 in 1961 to
    13,495 in 1981; and Regina's population increased elevenfold in two dec-
    ades, from 539 in 1961 to 6,575 in 1981. Put another way, the off-reserve
    "Registered Indian" population increased 81 per cent in the decade after
    1966. Peters, "Our City Indians" (2002), 78. As Mary Jane Norris and
    Stewart Clatworthy note, census and population statistics are notoriously
    unreliable: "Among the four different Aboriginal populations – First
    Nations, Registered and Non-Status Indians, Métis, and Inuit – Registered
    Indians are the only Aboriginal groups for whom reasonably consistent
    census data exist back to the 1960s." Norris and Clatworthy,
    "Urbanization and Migration Patterns" (2011), 16.

24 Peters, "Our City Indians," 75.
25 Quoted in Peters, "Aboriginal People" (1998), 249.
26 The National Indian Council, established in 1961, attempted to build
    a national network to promote unity and regional organizations. The
    council's leadership was largely urban and represented Métis, status, and
    non-status Indians with few reserve representatives. The subsequent clash
    of interests prompted its dissolution in 1968 and the creation of NIB and
    the Native Council of Canada for Métis and non-status Indians. Weaver,
    Making Canadian Indian Policy, 42–3.
27 Cardinal, *Unjust Society*, 1.
28 Weaver, *Making Canadian Indian Policy*, 199.
29 The occupation of Alcatraz between 1969 and 1971 provided a template
    for North American Indigenous activism. AIM led the seventy-one-day
    occupation of Wounded Knee in South Dakota in February 1973.
30 Ryan, *Wall of Words* (1978).
31 Rutherford, "Canada's Other Red Scare" (2011), 158.
32 Weaver, *Making Canadian Indian Policy*, 202; Rutherford, "Canada's
    Other Red Scare," 193.
33 Weaver, *Making Canadian Indian Policy*, 201.
34 "Five Years on an Indian Reserve," 1971, F825-2, Records of Ontario
    Planned Parenthood, B229874, AO.
35 Quoted in Anderson and Lawrence, *Strong Women Stories* (2003), 181.
36 Ibid., 177.
37 Magee, "For Home and Country" (2009), 27–49.
38 R.M. Connelly to regional director, 3 October 1972, RG10, 1996-97/250,
    box 9, file 601/24-5, LAC.
39 Barkaskas, "*Indian Voice*" (2009), 10–11.
40 See Indian Homemakers Association, 20 January 1981, RG10,
    acc. 1994-95/ 595, box 16, file E-6417-2254, pt. 1, LAC.
41 In 1984, with no further funding, the *Indian Voice* stopped publication;
    the BCIHA disbanded in the early 2000s. Barkaskas, "*Indian Voice*,"
    ii, 41.
42 Quoted in Barker, "Gender, Sovereignty," 130.
43 The two primary groups, Indian Rights for Indian Women (IRIW) and the
    Native Women's Association of Canada (NWAC), focused nationally on
    securing a repeal of the status provisions of the Indian Act. In the lawsuits
    mentioned earlier – *Lavell* (1973), *Bédard* (1972), and *Lovelace* (1981) –
    the women challenged the constitutionality and human rights compliance
    of the patrilineal criterion for status. Barker, "Gender, Sovereignty," 135–6.

44 Weaver, *Making Canadian Indian* Policy, 199.
45 Barker, "Gender, Sovereignty," 137.
46 Carlson and Steinhauer, *Disinherited Generations* (2013), 69, 70.
47 Glenn with Green, "Colleen Glenn," 237.
48 LaRocque, "Métis and Feminist," 66, 68.
49 Anderson, "Affirmations" (2010), 87.
50 Wiebe to professional staff, "Confidential, Family Planning Policy," LAC.
51 C.A. Bentley to Gentlemen, "Specimen Letter," 18 July 1973, RG29, acc. 1987-88/254, vol. 2, file 150-1-24, pt. 2, LAC.
52 G.C. Butler, regional director, to zone director, 20 July 1973, RG29, acc. 1987-88/254, vol. 2, file 150-1-24, pt. 2, LAC.
53 Regional director to senior consultant, Medical Services Branch, "Confidential," 5 October 1973, RG29, acc. 1987-88/254, vol. 2, file 150-1-24, pt. 2, LAC.
54 Native Women's Association of Manitoba, *Family Planning and Birth Control Methods* (Winnipeg: Native Women's Association of Manitoba, 1974; reprinted twice in 1975), Planned Parenthood Association collection, MG28, I 463, file 37.3, LAC.
55 "Five Years on an Indian Reserve," n.p.
56 W.G. Goldthorpe to director general, 6 February 1974, RG29, vol. 2870, file 851-1-5, pt. 3b, LAC.
57 The 1969 amended law limited the procedure to accredited hospitals with a three-doctor therapeutic abortion committee that ultimately decided women's fate. Rebick, *Ten Thousand Roses* (2005), 36.
58 Charles-E. Caron, assistant deputy minister, to Pierre Gravelle, assistant deputy minister, Health Programs, 16 June 1976, RG29, acc. 1996-97/698, box 53, file 6756-2-6, pt. 3, LAC.
59 Only Whitehorse, Charles Camsell, Sioux Lookout (in 1975), and Fort Qu'Appelle Indian Hospitals were accredited by 1976, but neither of the latter two performed abortions. Charles-E. Caron, assistant deputy minister, to Jean Lupien, deputy minister health, 28 April 1976, RG29, acc. 1996-97/698, box 53, file 6756-2-6, pt. 3, LAC.
60 A.E. Boehm, executive director, Charles Camsell Hospital, to J. Kirkbride, regional director, 4 May 1976, RG29, vol. 2954, file 851-3-13 pt. 5, LAC.
61 N.L. Fraser, regional director, Ontario region, to director general, 14 May 1976, RG29, vol. 2954, file 851-3-13 pt. 5, LAC.
62 Caron to Lupien, 28 April 1976, LAC.
63 Schoen, *Choice and Coercion* (2006), 21.

CHAPTER FOUR

1 Law Reform Commission of Canada (LRCC), "Protection of Life" (1979), 27.
2 Ibid., 29, 31.
3 For examples of this line of reasoning, see the interviews with disability activists (especially Nicola Fairbrother) collected at EugenicsArchive.ca, accessed 20 January 2018, http://eugenicsarchive.ca/discover/interviews.
4 For a comprehensive look at an Ontario facility, Huronia Regional Centre, see Simmons, *From Asylum to Welfare* (1982).
5 Correspondence re: Depo Provera in government facilities, Zarfas Files, 3.20B, Centre for Addiction and Mental Health Archives, Toronto (hereafter CAMH Archives).
6 On this topic, see, for example, Kluchin, *Fit to Be Tied*; Schoen, *Choice and Coercion*; and Kline, *Building a Better Race*.
7 Dyck, *Facing Eugenics*; Malacrida, *Special Hell*; McLaren, *Our Own Master Race*; Grekul, "Social Construction" (2002); Caulfield and Robertson, "Eugenic Policies in Alberta" (1996); Chapman, "Early Eugenics Movements" (1977); Devereux, *Growing a Race* (2005); Harris-Zsovan, *Eugenics and the Firewall* (2010); Muir, *Whisper Past* (2014); Samson, "Eugenics in the Community."
8 Braslow, *Mental Ills* (1997); Stern, "From Legislation to Lived Experience" (2011); Weindling, *Victims and Survivors*; Turda, ed., *East-Central European Eugenics* (2015).
9 Alberta, Institute of Law Research and Reform, *Competence and Human Reproduction* (1989), 2. For the 1968 Alberta report, see Blair, *Mental Health in Alberta* (1969), 267.
10 Blair, *Mental Health in Alberta*, 267.
11 Robert Welch, provincial secretary, to W. Darcy McKeough, MPP, memo, 1973, CR144621, AO.
12 Hal Jackson, secretariat for social development, to the Hon. R. Welch, QC, provincial secretary for social development, memo, CR144621, AO.
13 Emily Murphy, *Lethbridge Herald*, 26 June [1932], n.p. (also published as "Overpopulation and Birth Control," *Vancouver Sun*, 1 October 1932, n.p.), Legislative Scrapbooks, microfilm, Edmonton City Archives.
14 LRCC, "Protection of Life," 107, 116.
15 Stan Oziewicz, "Retarded Children Sterilized Illegally, Guardian Contends," *Globe and Mail*, 12 December 1978, 1.
16 Ibid., 2

17 Ibid., 2.
18 "Sterilization of Retarded Discussed," *Globe and Mail*, 7 December 1979.
19 Ibid.
20 "Ontario Sterilization Ban Extended" (1979), 1293.
21 Dr Norman Brown, Canadian Medical Protective Association (CMPA), to Dr Ian Burgess, vice-president, Salvation Army Grace Hospital, Calgary, 2 November 1978, 1, Grace Hospital-011, Calgary Health Services Archives.
22 Desjardins, "Sexualized Body" (2012), 79.
23 Zarfas quoted in David Luginbuhl, letter to *Canadian Family Physician*, 1979, GRA-011, 1293, Calgary Health Services Archives.
24 Wolfensberger, *Principle of Normalization* (1972).
25 "Fertility a Problem in Residences for the Retarded, Doctor Says," *Globe and Mail*, 8 April 1978, 4.
26 "'Sterilize Her' Retarded Girl's Mother Urged," *Globe and Mail*, n.d., clippings file, Zarfas Files, CAMH Archives.
27 Green and Paul, "Parenthood and the Mentally Retarded" (1974), 118.
28 Goffman, *Asylums* (1961).
29 "Sterilisation Ban Is Sought," *Calgary Herald*, 9 December 1979, B3.
30 "Fight on Forced Sterilization Is Raging in Canada," editorial, *Medical Tribune World Service*, 14 February 1979, 1.
31 "Canada Acts to End Sterilization Abuse," editorial, *Medical Tribune World Service*, 14 February 1979, 15.
32 John Emslie to "Whom it may concern," 12 February 1979, 1, Zarfas Files, 9.13, CAMH Archives.
33 Ibid., 1.
34 Ibid., 2.
35 Ibid., 2.
36 Ibid., 3.
37 "MDs Could be Charged for Sterilizing Retarded," no source listed, n.d., clippings file, Zarfas Files, CAMH Archives.
38 Zarfas, "Preliminary Report on Survery of Parental Attitudes," 1978, Zarfas Files, 6.25, CAMH Archives.
39 "Parents of Retarded Favor Sterilization" *Hamilton Spectator*, 26 March 1980, n.p., clippings file, Zarfas Files, 9.10, CAMH Archives.
40 Dr Norman Brown to Dr Ian Burgess, 2 November 1978, 1, Zarfas Files, CAMH Archives.
41 "Guidelines for Sterilization of Mentally Retarded Persons" *Ontario Medical Review*, July 1980, 346, Zarfas Files, 9.10, CAMH Archives.

42 Brown to Burgess, 2 November 1978, 1.

43 Kathleen Rex, "Hospital Refused Sterilization, Parents of Retarded Girl Complain," *Globe and Mail*, 8 February 1979.

44 Ibid.

45 "Protect Mentally Ill from Sterilization, Says Law Reform Commission," *Calgary Herald*, 9 December 1979, B3.

46 Dyck, *Facing Eugenics*, 223.

47 Dooley, "End of the Asylum" (2011).

48 Donald Zarfas to Gilbert Sharp, chairman of the Interministerial [*sic*] Committee on Consents, re: Committee on Sterilization of the Mentally Retarded, 12 February 1979, 1, Zarfas Files, 9.13, CAMH Archives.

49 Donald Zarfas, "Sterilization of Mentally Defective Females," notes for an address, 1978, 1, Zarfas Files, 2.8, CAMH Archives.

50 Ibid.

51 Schoen, *Choice and Coercion*; Solinger, *Reproductive Politics* (2013).

52 Zarfas, "Sterilization of Mentally Deficient Females," 1.

53 Zarfas, "Sterilization of Mentally Deficient Females," 2, 5.

54 Ladd-Taylor, "Contraception or Eugenics?"

55 For more examples that challenge these boundaries, see "Our Stories," Eugenicsarchive.ca, n.d., accessed 20 January 2018, http://eugenicsarchive. ca/discover/our-stories. Some of the contemporary examples in this collection reveal the ways that elements of newgenics continue to frame ideas about capable parenthood, as well as the notion that restricting these people from parenting serves to prevent mental disorder and dependence. In particular, see the stories by Candace, Eric, and Velvet.

56 David Luginbuhl to Lieutenant Colonel D. Routly, Women's Social Services secretary, Salvation Army Headquarters, 16 May 1983, 1, Calgary Health Services Archives.

57 Zarfas, "Report to the Ontario Medical Association on the Sterilization of Mentally-Retarded Persons," 1978, 5, Zarfas Files, CAMH Archives.

58 Dorothy Lipovenko, "OHIP Pays for Sterilization of Retarded," *Globe and Mail*, 13 August 1980, 15. For a thorough account of travelling for abortion, see Sethna and David, eds., *Abortion across Borders*.

59 Lipovenko, "OHIP Pays," 15.

60 Alberta, Institute of Law Research and Reform, *Competence and Human Reproduction*, 2.

61 Alberta, Institute of Law Research and Reform, *Sterilization Decisions* (1988), 1.

62 Tomes, "Patient as a Policy Factor" (2006).

CHAPTER FIVE

1 Revie, "More Than Just Boots" (2006).
2 McLaren and McLaren, *Bedroom and the State*; Dyck, *Facing Eugenics*, chap. 1. See also Katz, Engelman, and Hajo, eds., *Selected Papers of Margaret Sanger*.
3 Shropshire, "What's a Guy To Do?"
4 Stern, *Eugenic Nation*, xiv.
5 See especially Shorter, *History of Women's Bodies* (1982).
6 Barnes, *Conceiving Masculinity* (2014), 7.
7 Shropshire, "What's a Guy To Do?," 167; see also Connell and Messerschmidt, "Hegemonic Masculinity" (2005).
8 Barnes, *Conceiving Masculinity*, 163.
9 Vasectomy continues to be underused by American men from racialized minority communities. Borrero et al., "Low Rates of Vasectomy" (2010); Fransoo et al., "Social Gradients" (2013).
10 From 1976 to 1986, more than 1.3 million Canadians were surgically sterilized; there were more than twice as many tubal ligations (934,647) than vasectomies (458,378) in those eleven years. But in 1986 in Newfoundland there were more vasectomies (1,292) than tubal ligations (1,050) and in Quebec there were nearly equal numbers of tubal ligation (19,818) and vasectomy (19,491). Alderman and Gee, "Sterilization" (1989).
11 Dr W.J. Hannah, "The Role of Surgical Procedures in Family Planning," *Bulletin: The Council for Social Service*, June 1966; Proceedings of a Symposium for Clergy and Physicians Counselling in Family Planning, 20 April 1966, Planned Parenthood Federation, both in MG28, I 463 41, file 41.12, LAC.
12 A.R. Kaufman, "Progress of Birth Control in Canada," 2 December 1969, MG28, I 463 40, file 40-39, 1969, LAC.
13 Revie, "More Than Just Boots," 128–9.
14 Herc Munro, "The Eccentric World of Alvin Ratz Kaufman," *Executive*, April 1962, GA58: Parents' Information Bureau series 3, file 36, University of Waterloo Archives.
15 McLaren, *Our Own Master Race*, 115.
16 Kaufman to Association for Voluntary Sterilization, 8 October 1968; Kaufman to John Rague, 28 October 1968, both in Records of the Association of Voluntary Sterilization (AVS), RC50, folder 27, Social Welfare History Archives, University of Minnesota (hereafter SW15); Revie, "More Than Just Boots," 129.

17 Weber to Miss Armes, Human Betterment Association, New York, 1 September 1954, AVS, RC 44, "Parents' Information Bureau 1955–1964" folder, SW 15.

18 "Interview Report between AR Kaufman and Miss IH Armes, 22 Aug 1952," AVS, RC 44, "Parents' Information Bureau 1955–1964" folder, SW 15.

19 Ruth Proskauer Smith to Kaufman, 1 May 1957, AVS, RC 56, folder 94, SW 15.

20 Kluchin, *Fit to be Tied*, 28.

21 Ibid., 34; John Rague to A.R Kaufman, 19 December 1969, AVS, RC 50, folder 27, SW 15.

22 Kaufman to Rague, 15 December 1969, AVS, RC 50, folder 27, SW 15.

23 Kaufman to Rague, 1 June 1966, AVS, RC 50, folder 27, SW 15.

24 Kaufman to AVS, 19 September 1973, AVS, RC 50, folder 27, SW 15.

25 Kaufman to Human Betterment Association, 8 March 1960, AVS, RC 44, SW 15.

26 Bruner, "Safe, Certain" (1961), 12.

27 "Male Sterilization," *Maclean's* (1962).

28 "Vasectomy," *Chatelaine* (1963).

29 Kaufman to Human Betterment Association, 3 May 1963, AVS, RC 56, folder 94, SW 15.

30 "Looking Back on the Birth Control Movement," *Close-Up*, CBC Television, aired 11 November 1962, CBC Digital Archives, https://www.cbc.ca/archives/entry/looking-back-on-the-birth-control-movement.

31 Kaufman to Association for Voluntary Sterilization, 6 January 1969, AVS, RC 50, folder 27, SW 15. Television cameras were not flattering for the bald, eighty-four-year-old Kaufman, who spoke with a stutter.

32 Kaufman to Mrs R.P. Smith, 4 July 1962, AVS, RC 56, folder 94, SW 15.

33 Kaufman to Rague, 18 August 1969, AVS, RC 50, folder 27, SW 15.

34 Kaufman to Rague, AVS, 15 March 1971, AVS, RC 50, folder 27, SW 15.

35 "Compulsory Vasectomies at 16 Advocated by Feminist Sociologist," *Globe and Mail*, 19 April 1968, 9.

36 Ibid.

37 "Doctors Recommend Vasectomy Legislation," *Globe and Mail*, 13 May 1967, 11.

38 "Now It's V for Vasectomy – and It's Becoming a Sign Seen Often," *Toronto Star*, 2 February 1974, f7.

39 Richards, "Vasectomy" (1973).

40 "V for Vasectomy," *Toronto Star*, f7.

41 Grindstaff and Ebanks, "Male Sterilization" (1973). Grindstaff was president of the London chapter of Planned Parenthood Ontario. "Community

Health through Family Planning: An Examination of Family Planning in Ontario," September 1973, RG 10-26, B 110622, AO.

42 "Voluntary Sterilization – the Surest Way to Avoid Unwanted Pregnancies," Planned Parenthood Ottawa Newsletter, May 1975, F 825-5, B 229874, AO.

43 "Population Control – Challenge Facing Our Society," *Toronto Star*, 19 February 1973, 9.

44 Wolfers and Wolfers, "Vasectomania," 197, 198, 199.

45 David Lancashire, "Vasectomy: Gaining Fast in the Birth-Control Race," *Globe and Mail*, 28 May 1977, 10. The genre continues in the twenty-first century: for example, "Men – Don't Be Squeamish, Have the Balls to Have a Vasectomy," *Guardian*, 21 October 2016; "Man Up Guys – You're a Snip Away from Being Heroes," *Guardian*, 24 June 2017.

46 Lancashire, "Vasectomy," 10.

47 Ibid.

48 In 1977 in Ontario, the tubal ligation rate (per 1,000 women aged 15 to 44) was 19.7; the vasectomy rate (per 1,000 men aged 20 to 49) was 8.6. Marcil-Gratton and Lapierre-Adamcyk, "Sterilization in Quebec" (1983), 77.

49 McClure in Lancashire, "Vasectomy," 10.

50 Wolfers and Wolfers, "Vasectomania," 199; Simon Population Trust, *Vasectomy*.

51 Lancashire, "Vasectomy," 10.

52 Livingstone, "Vasectomy" (1971), 1065.

53 Shropshire, "What's a Guy To Do?," 169–70.

54 Richards, "Vasectomy."

55 Marcil-Gratton and Lapierre-Adamcyk, "Sterilization in Quebec," 75, 76.

56 Ibid.

57 The vasectomy rate is calculated per 1,000 men aged twenty to forty-nine; the tubal ligation rate is per 1,000 women aged fifteen to forty-four. Ibid., 77.

58 Statistics for Newfoundland were available only for 1982 to 1986; statistics for the Territories were not available. Alderman and Gee, "Sterilization," 645, 646, 647.

59 Quoted in Alderman, "Vasectomies" (1988), 1751.

60 "V for Vasectomy," *Toronto Star*, f7.

61 Alderman, "Vasectomies."

62 Alderman and Gee, "Sterilization."

63 The other countries were Bhutan, New Zealand, the Netherlands, and Great Britain. Pile and Barone, "Demographics of Vasectomy" (2009).

64 Fransoo et al., "Social Gradients." In the United States a similar link exists between social and economic advantage and vasectomy. Eeckhaut and Sweeney, "Perplexing Links" (2016).

CHAPTER SIX

1 Balcom, *Traffic in Babies* (2011); Dubinsky, *Babies without Borders* (2010).
2 Blair, "'Babies Needn't Follow'" (2020).
3 Powell and Deber, "Number of Pregnancies" (1982), 493.
4 Ibid, 495.
5 Statistics Canada, *Therapeutic Abortions, 1975* (1977), 70–1.
6 Statistics Canada, *Therapeutic Abortions, 1977: Advance Information* (1978), 12.
7 Ibid., 6.
8 We are grateful to Matthew DeCloedt for collecting these statistics for us.
9 Statistics Canada, *Therapeutic Abortions, 1976* (1979), 37.
10 Ibid., 82.
11 Canada, *Some Facts about Therapeutic Abortions in Canada, 1970–1982* (1984), 18. See also Canada, *Selected Therapeutic Abortion Statistics, 1970–1991* (1994), 17–18.
12 Statistics Canada, *Therapeutic Abortions, 1975* (1977), 25.
13 Ibid.
14 Statistics Canada, *Therapeutic Abortions, 1976* (1979), 33.
15 Holz, *Birth Control Clinic* (2012).
16 Patton, "We Were Having Conversations" (2013).
17 Stevenson, "Intimate Integration."
18 Statistics Canada, *Therapeutic Abortions, 1973* (1974), 6.
19 Statistics Canada, *Therapeutic Abortions, 1972* (1973), 6; Sethna, "All Aboard?" (2011), 90–1; Palmer, "Lonely, Tragic."
20 Statistics Canada, *Therapeutic Abortions, 1972*, 36–7.
21 "Community Responses, Needs and Priorities in Family Planning," First Provincial Conference, Family Planning Association of BC, 21–24 May 1973, 37, GR2698, BC Archives, Victoria (hereafter BCA).
22 Ibid.
23 Ibid., 5.
24 G.R.F. Elliot (MD), deputy minister of health, to Miss Ruth Taylor, ActionLine, *The Province*, Vancouver, re: Mrs A. Charles, Kelowna, 27 April 1973, GR 2698, BCA.

25 Dennis Cocke, minister of health, to Mrs R.J. Hawkins, Powell River, "Family Planning & Abortion & Miscellaneous," 1974, GR 2698, box 2, BCA.

26 Letter from Vancouver Women's Health Clinic, 146 East 18th, Vancouver, 26 July 1973, GR 2698, box 2, BCA.

27 Family Planning Association Newsletter, 30 June 1973, 3, BCA.

28 See Comacchio, *Nations Are Built of Babies* (1993). Comacchio reminds us that this paternalism has a long history of public health campaigns that centre around protecting women who are considered incapable of protecting themselves.

29 Nova Scotia Department of Health Family Planning Project, "Director's Report," 1981, 4, Health and Welfare Grant #4458-2-1, RG25, vol. 657, no. 8, Family Planning Project collection, Nova Scotia Archives, Halifax (hereafter NSA).

30 Canadian Abortion Rights Action League (CARAL), Halifax Chapter, *Telling Our Secrets: Abortion Stories from Nova Scotia*, comp. Nancy Bowes (Halifax: CARAL, 1990), 1, V/F V.348 no. 7, NSA.

31 Ibid.

32 Quoted in Nova Scotia Department of Health Family Planning Project, "Director's Report," 4, reprinted from Planned Parenthood Federation of America, *Eleven Million Teenagers* (New York, 1976).

33 Nova Scotia Department of Health Family Planning Project, "Director's Report," 7.

34 Ibid, 1–3.

35 Coral Cowell, "An Exploration of the Limitations of Contraception," unpublished research paper, n.d., 37, RG25, vol. 657, no. 8, Family Planning Project collection, NSA.

36 Untitled report, n.d., 4, RG25, vol. 657, no. 8, Family Planning Project collection, NSA.

37 Agnes Higgins, Nutrition Conference, New Glasgow, April 1979, RG25, vol. 657, no. 8, Family Planning Project collection, NSA.

38 Susan MacDonnell (Dept. of Social Services, Social Research and Planning Division), "Vulnerable Mothers, Vulnerable Children: A Follow-Up Study of the Unmarried Mother Who Keeps Her Child," [1974], 2, RG25, vol. 657, no. 8, Family Planning Project collection, NSA.

39 Schlesinger, *Family Planning in Canada* (1974), n.p., quoted in untitled report, 5, Family Planning Project collection, NSA.

40 Schlesinger, ed., *Family Planning in Canada*.

41 Untitled report, 5, Family Planning Project collection, NSA

42 CARAL, Halifax Chapter, *Telling Our Secrets*, 1.

43 Ibid., 2.
44 Ibid., 12.
45 Ibid., 28.
46 Ibid., 13.
47 Ibid., 41.
48 Ibid., 16.
49 Ibid., 20–1.
50 For more on this book and its influence, see Kline, *Bodies of Knowledge* (2010).
51 CARAL, Halifax Chapter, *Telling Our Secrets*, 35.
52 Ibid., 44.
53 Ibid., 38–9; emphases in original.
54 Ibid., 28.
55 "Routine Prescription of Contraceptives Opposed: Unmarried Teen-Age Girls Suffer Depression, Sense of Worthlessness, after Abortion, MD Says," *Globe and Mail*, 1 December 1971, 11.
56 Joan Hollobon, "Patients May Face Problems as Adults: A Third of Abortions on Adolescents Go Wrong: MD," *Globe and Mail*, 29 January 1972, 13.
57 For a good review of these trials, see *The Pill* (2003).
58 Watkins, *On the Pill*, 43, 88.
59 "Pill Advocate Claims Pregnancy Causes 15 Times More Deaths," *Globe and Mail*, 26 February 1970, W8.
60 "The Penalty of Pregnancy," *Globe and Mail*, 15 March 1971, 6.
61 Joan Hollobon, "Teen-Agers Who Participate in Sex Told to Use Contraceptives," *Globe and Mail*, 21 October 1972, 14.
62 "Crisis Needs across Canada," 36, appendix 2 in *Community Responses, Needs and Priorities*, GR 2698, BCA.
63 Mary F. Bishop, "Welcome and Conference Concept," 22 May 1973, 5, in *Community Responses, Needs and Priorities*, GR 2698, BCA.
64 "Feature: Teen Marriages," *Kainai News*, 2 February 1978, 8.
65 Elliot to Taylor, 27 April 1973, 2, BCA.
66 Ibid.
67 Mr Mainguy to Minister's Office, 13 February 1975, GR 2698, BCA.

CONCLUSION

1 Martin Regg Cohn, "Doug Ford's 'Father Knows Best' Sex-Ed Strategy Places Ideology over Biology," *Toronto Star*, 5 September 2018.
2 Shiva and Shiva, "Population and Environment" (1993), 20.

3 Ibid.

4 Ibid., 21.

5 Statistics Canada, "Population Growth," in *Aboriginal Statistics at a Glance*, 89-645-x, last modified 30 November 2015, https://www150. statcan.gc.ca/n1/pub/89-645-x/2010001/growth-pop-croissance-eng.htm. Growth rate is defined as the percentage of increase in the population between two specified periods of time.

6 See, for example, Jason Warick, "Indigenous Population Growing Rapidly in Sask.: Stats Can," CBC News, 25 October 2017, https://www.cbc.ca/ news/canada/saskatoon/fn-population-growing-fast-1.4371422.

7 The issues of genetic screening and fertility treatments are beyond the scope of this book; for examples of this history in the United States, see Stillwell, "Interpreting the Genetic Revolution" (2013); and Cowan, *Heredity and Hope* (2008).

8 "China," Climate Action Tracker, accessed 24 September 2018, https:// climateactiontracker.org/countries/china/.

9 See Erin Duffin, "Average Life Expectancy in Africa for Those Born in 2019, by Gender and Region," Statista, 20 September 2019, https://www. statista.com/statistics/274511/life-expectancy-in-africa/.

Bibliography

ARCHIVES CONSULTED

Archives of Ontario
British Columbia Archives
British Columbia Statutes
Centre for Addiction and Mental Health Archives
CBC Archives
Glenbow Archives
Library and Archives Canada
Nova Scotia Archives
Provincial Archives of Alberta
Provincial Archives of Saskatchewan
Yukon Archives

NEWSPAPERS

Calgary Herald
Edmonton Journal
Globe and Mail
Kainai News
Leader Post (Regina)
Peninsula Times (Sechelt, BC)
Star Phoenix (Saskatoon)
Toronto Star

LEGAL SOURCES

An Act Respecting Sexual Sterilization, S.B.C. 1933, c 59 (British Columbia).

Alberta. Institute of Law Research and Reform. *Competence and Human Reproduction.* Report No. 52. Edmonton, February 1989.

Alberta. Institute of Law Research and Reform. *Sterilization Decisions: Minors and Mentally Incompetent Adults.* Report for Discussion No. 6. Edmonton, March 1988.

Attorney General of Canada v. Lavell, [1974] S.C.R. 1349.

Bédard v. Isaac et al., [1972] 2 O.R. 391.

Criminal Law Amendment Act 1968–69, S.C. 1968–69, c. 38.

E. (Mrs.) v. Eve, [1986] 2 S.C.R. 388.

Indian Act, R.S.C., 1906, c. 81, s. 142.

Indian Act, R.S.C., 1985, c. I-5.

Sandra Lovelace v. Canada, Communication No. 24/1977: Canada 30/07/81, UN Doc. CCPR/C/13/D/24/1977.

Sexual Sterilization Act, S.A. 1928, c. 37 (Alberta).

SECONDARY SOURCES

Alderman, Philip. "Vasectomies: Motivations and Attitudes of Physicians-as-Patients." *Canadian Family Physician* 34 (1988): 1749–52.

Alderman, Philip M., and Ellen M. Gee. "Sterilization: Canadian Choices." *Canadian Medical Association Journal* 140, no. 6 (1989): 645–9.

Anderson, Kim. "Affirmations of an Indigenous Feminist." In *Indigenous Women and Feminism: Politics, Activism, Culture*, ed. Cheryl Suzack, Shari M. Huhndorf, Jeanne Perreault, and Jean Barman, 81–91. Vancouver: UBC Press, 2010.

– *A Recognition of Being: Reconstructing Native Womanhood.* Toronto: Sumach Press, 2000.

Anderson, Kim, and Bonita Lawrence. *Strong Women Stories: Native Vision and Community Survival.* Toronto: Sumach Press, 2003.

Appleby, Brenda Margaret. *Responsible Parenthood: Decriminalizing Contraception in Canada.* Toronto: University of Toronto Press, 1999.

Backhouse, Constance. *Prejudice and Petticoats: Women and Law in Nineteenth-Century Canada.* Toronto: Osgood Society, 1991.

Baillargeon, Denyse. *Babies for the Nation: The Medicalization of Motherhood in Quebec, 1910–1970.* Waterloo: Wilfrid Laurier University Press, 2009.

Balcom, Karen. *The Traffic in Babies: Cross-Border Adoption and Baby-Selling between the United States and Canada, 1930–1972*. Toronto: University of Toronto Press, 2011.

Barkaskas, Patricia Miranda. "*The Indian Voice*: Centering Women in the Gendered Politics of Indigenous Nationalism in BC, 1969–1984." MA thesis, University of British Columbia, 2009.

Barker, Joanne. "Gender, Sovereignty, and the Discourse of Rights in Native Women's Activism." *Meridians: Feminism, Race, Transnationalism* 7, no. 1 (2006): 127–61.

Barnes, Liberty Walther. *Conceiving Masculinity: Male Infertility, Medicine, and Identity*. Philadelphia: Temple University Press, 2014.

Bashford, Alison. *Global Population: History, Geopolitics, and Life on Earth*. New York: Columbia University Press, 2014.

Bashford, Alison, and Philippa Levine, eds. *The Oxford Handbook of the History of Eugenics*. Oxford: Oxford University Press, 2010.

Blacker, C.P. "The International Planned Parenthood Federation: Some Aspects of Its History." *Eugenics Review* 56, no. 3 (1964): 135–42.

Blair, Megan. "'Babies Needn't Follow': Birth Control and Abortion Policy Activism at the University of Waterloo and Waterloo Lutheran University, 1965–74." Advance online article. *Canadian Bulletin of Medical History* (20 March 2020). https://doi.org/10.3138/cbmh.355-052019.

Blair, W.R.N. *Mental Health in Alberta: A Report on the Alberta Mental Health Study, 1968*. Edmonton: Human Resources Research and Development, Executive Council, Government of Alberta, 1969.

Blake, Raymond. *From Rights to Needs: A History of Family Allowances in Canada, 1929–92*. Vancouver: UBC Press, 2009.

Bock, Gisela. "Racism and Sexism in Nazi Germany: Motherhood, Compulsory Sterilization and the State." *Signs* 8, no. 31 (1983): 400–21.

Borrero, Sonya, Charity G. Moore, Mitchell D. Creinin, and Said A. Ibrahim. "Low Rates of Vasectomy among Minorities." *American Journal of Men's Health* 4, no. 3 (2010): 243–49.

Boyer, Yvonne. "First Nations, Métis and Inuit Health and the Law: A Framework for the Future." LLD thesis, University of Ottawa, 2011.

Braslow, Joel. *Mental Ills and Bodily Cures: Psychiatric Treatment in the First Half of the Twentieth Century*. Berkeley: University of California Press, 1997.

Briggs, Laura. "Discourses of 'Forced Sterilization' in Puerto Rico: The Problem with the Speaking Subaltern." *Differences: A Journal of Feminist Cultural Studies* 10, no. 2 (1998). Gale Academic OneFile.

– *Reproducing Empire: Race, Sex, Science, and US Imperialism in Puerto Rico.* Berkeley: University of California Press, 2002.

Bruner, Arnold. "The Safe, Certain Birth-Control Method That Doctors Won't Talk About." *Maclean's,* 12 August 1961.

Bulmer, Michael. *Francis Galton: Pioneer of Heredity and Biometry.* Baltimore: Johns Hopkins University Press, 2003.

Campbell, Lara, Dominique Clément, and Gregory Kealey, eds. *Debating Dissent: Canada and the Sixties.* Toronto: University of Toronto Press, 2012.

Canada. Parliament. House of Commons. *Debates.* 28th Parl., 1st Sess., vol. 7 (1969).

– *Debates.* 28th Parl., 1st Sess., vol. 8 (1969).

– *Debates.* 28th Parl., 3rd Sess., vol. 1 (1970).

Canada. Royal Commission on the Status of Women. *Report.* Ottawa, 7 December 1970.

Cardinal, Harold. *The Unjust Society: The Tragedy of Canada's Indians.* Edmonton: M.G. Hurtig, 1969.

Carlson, Nellie, and Kathleen Steinhauer. *Disinherited Generations: Our Struggle to Reclaim Treaty Rights for First Nations Women and Their Descendants.* Edmonton: University of Alberta Press, 2013.

Caulfield, Tim, and Gerald Robertson. "Eugenic Policies in Alberta: From the Systematic to the Systemic?" *Alberta Law Review* 35, no. 1 (1996): 59–79.

Chapman, Terry. "Early Eugenics Movements in Western Canada." *Alberta History* 25, no. 4 (1977): 9–17.

Chisholm, Christine. "The Curious Case of Thalidomide and the Absent Eugenics Clause in Canada's Amended Abortion Law of 1969." *Canadian Bulletin of Medical History* 33, no. 2 (2016): 493–516.

Clow, Barbara. "'An Illness of Nine Months' Duration': Pregnancy and Thalidomide Use in Canada and the United States." In *Women, Health, and Nation: Canada and the United States since 1945,* ed. Georgina Feldberg, Molly Ladd-Taylor, Alison Li, and Kathryn McPherson, 45–66. Montreal and Kingston: McGill-Queen's University Press, 2003.

Coates, Ken. *Best Left as Indians: Native-White Relations in the Yukon Territory, 1840–1973.* Montreal and Kingston: McGill-Queen's University Press, 1991.

Comacchio, Cynthia. *Nations Are Built of Babies: Saving Ontario's Mothers and Children, 1900–1940.* Montreal and Kingston: McGill-Queen's University Press, 1993.

Connell, R.W., and James W. Messerschmidt. "Hegemonic Masculinity: Rethinking the Concept." *Gender and Society* 19, no. 6 (2005): 829–59.

Connelly, Matthew. *Fatal Misconception: The Struggle to Control World Population*. Cambridge, MA: Harvard University Press, 2008.

– "Seeing beyond the State: The Population Control Movement and the Problem of Sovereignty." *Past and Present*, no. 193 (2006): 197–233.

Cowan, Ruth Schwartz. *Heredity and Hope: The Case for Genetic Screening*. Cambridge, MA: Harvard University Press, 2008.

Deighton, Alex. "The Nature of Eugenic Thought and the Limits of Eugenic Practice in Interwar Saskatchewan." In *Eugenics at the Edges of Empire: New Zealand, Australia, Canada, and South Africa*, ed. Diane Paul, John Stenhouse, and Hamish Spencer, 63–84. Gewerbestrasse, Switzerland: Palgrave Macmillan, 2018.

Desjardins, Michel. "La construction anthropologique des problèmes sociaux, l'exemple de la déficience intellectuelle." In *Nouvelles configurations des problèmes sociaux et l'intervention*, ed. Robert Mayer and Henri Dorvil, 175–90. Sainte-Foy: Presses de l'Université du Québec, Sainte-Foy, 2001.

– "The Sexualized Body of the Child: Parents and the Politics of 'Voluntary' Sterilization of People Labeled Intellectually Disabled." In *Sex and Disability*, ed. R. McRuer and A. Mollow, 67–85. Durham: Duke University Press, 2012. PDF.

Devereux, Cecily. *Growing a Race: Nellie L. McClung and the Fiction of Eugenic Feminism*. Montreal and Kingston: McGill-Queen's University Press, 2005.

Dodds, Donald J. *Voluntary Male Sterilization*. Toronto: Damian Press, 1970.

Dooley, Chris. "The End of the Asylum (Town): Community Responses to the Depopulation and Closure of the Saskatchewan Hospital, Weyburn." *Histoire Sociale* 44, no. 88 (2011): 331–54.

Dorr, Gregory Michael. *Segregation's Science: Eugenics and Society in Virginia*. Charlottesville: University of Virginia Press, 2008.

Dowbiggin, Ian. *The Sterilization Movement and Global Fertility in the Twentieth Century*. New York: Oxford University Press, 2008.

Dubinsky, Karen. *Babies without Borders: Adoption and Migration across the Americas*. New York: New York University Press, 2010.

Dunphy, Catherine. *Morgentaler: A Difficult Hero*. Toronto: Wiley, 2003.

Dyck, Erika. "Abortion and Birth Control on the Canadian Prairies: Feminists, Catholics, and Family Values in the 1970s." In Stettner, Burnett, and Hay, eds., *Abortion*, 74–94.

– "Eugenics in Canada: Choice, Coercion and Context." In *Eugenics at the Edges of Empire: New Zealand, Australia, Canada, and South Africa*, ed. Diane Paul, John Stenhouse, and Hamish Spencer, 41–62. Gewerbestrasse, Switzerland: Palgrave Macmillan, 2018.

– *Facing Eugenics: Reproduction, Sterilization, and the Politics of Choice.* Toronto: University of Toronto Press, 2013.

– "Sterilization and Birth Control in the Shadow of Eugenics: Married, Middle-Class Women in Alberta, 1930–1960s." *Canadian Bulletin of Medical History* 31, no. 1 (2014): 165–87.

Eeckhaut, Mieke C.W., and Megan M. Sweeney. "The Perplexing Links between Contraceptive Sterilization and (Dis)advantage in Ten Low-Fertility Countries." *Population Studies* 70, no. 1 (2016): 39–58.

Egan, Carolyn, and Linda Gardner. "Reproductive Freedom: The Ontario Coalition for Abortion Clinics and the Campaign to Overturn the Federal Abortion Law." In Stettner, ed., *Without Apology*, 131–8.

Ehrlich, Paul. *The Population Bomb.* New York: Sierra Club/Ballatine Books, 1968.

Feldberg, Georgina. "On the Cutting Edge: Science and Obstetrical Practice in a Women's Hospital, 1945–1960." In *Women, Health, and Nation: Canada and the United States since 1945*, ed. Georgina Feldberg, Molly Ladd-Taylor, Alison Li, and Kathryn McPherson, 123–43. Montreal and Kingston: McGill-Queen's University Press, 2003.

Fleming, Meredith, and Terrence C.R. Joyce. "Elective Sterilization of the Human Male (Vasectomy)." *Canadian Hospital* 445, no. 6 (1968): 1–3.

Foucault, Michel. *The Birth of Biopolitics: Lectures at the Collège de France, 1978–1979.* Translated by Graham Burchell. Edited by Michel Senellart. London: Palgrave Macmillan, 2008.

– *Discipline and Punish: The Birth of the Prison.* Translated by Alan Sheridan. New York: Pantheon, 1977.

– *Madness and Civilization: A History of Insanity in the Age of Reason.* Translated by Richard Howard. London: Routledge Classics, 2001.

Fransoo, Randall, Jill Bucklaschuk, Heather Prior, Elaine Burland, Daniel Chateau, Patricia Martens, and The Need To Know Team. "Social Gradients in Surgical Sterilization Rates: Opposing Patterns for Males and Females." *Journal of Obstetrics and Gynaecology Canada* 35, no. 5 (2013): 454–60.

Glenn, Colleen, with Joyce Green. "Colleen Glenn: A Metis Feminist in Indian Rights for Indian Women, 1973–1979." In Green, ed., *Making Space*, 233–40.

Goffman, Erving. *Asylums: Essays on the Social Situation of Mental Patients and Other Inmates.* Garden City, NY: Anchor Books, 1961.

Green, Bernard, and Rena Paul. "Parenthood and the Mentally Retarded." *University of Toronto Law Journal* 24, no. 2 (1974): 117–25.

Green, Joyce, ed. *Making Space for Indigenous Feminism.* Halifax: Fernwood, 2007.

– "Taking Account of Aboriginal Feminism," in Green, ed., *Making Space,* 20–32.

Grekul, Jana. "Social Construction of the 'Feeble-Minded Threat.'" Ph.D. diss., University of Alberta, 2002.

Grindstaff, Carl, and G. Edward Ebanks. "Male Sterilization as a Contraceptive Method in Canada: An Empirical Study." *Population Studies* 27, no. 3 (1973): 443–55.

Gurr, Barbara. *Reproductive Justice: The Politics of Health Care for Native American Women.* New Brunswick, NJ: Rutgers University Press, 2015.

Hansen, Randall, and Desmond King. *Sterilized by the State: Eugenics, Race, and the Population Scare in Twentieth-Century North America.* Cambridge: Cambridge University Press, 2013.

Hardin, Garrett. "1960: The World Rediscovers Malthus." In *Population Evolution and Birth Control: A Collage of Controversial Readings,* ed. Garrett Hardin, 46–7. San Francisco: W.H. Freeman, 1964.

Harris, Alana., ed. *The Schism of '68: Catholicism, Contraception and 'Humanae Vitae' in Europe, 1945–1975.* London: Palgrave Macmillan, 2016.

Harris-Zsovan, Jane. *Eugenics and the Firewall: Canada's Nasty Little Secret.* Winnipeg: J.G. Shillingford, 2010.

Haynes, Jessica. "The Great Emancipator? The Impact of the Birth-Control Pill on Married Women in English Canada, 1960–1980." Ph.D. diss., Carleton University, 2012.

Holz, Rose. *The Birth Control Clinic in a Marketplace World.* Rochester, NY: University of Rochester Press, 2012.

Huxley, Aldous. *Brave New World.* London, UK: Chatto & Windus, 1932.

– *Brave New World Revisited.* New York, NY: Harper & Row, 1958.

Igartua, José. *The Other Quiet Revolution: National Identities in English Canada, 1945–71.* Vancouver: UBC Press, 2006.

Ing, Rosalyn. "Canada's Indian Residential Schools and Their Impacts on Mothering." In Lavell-Harvard and Corbiere Lavell, eds., *"Until Our Hearts Are on the Ground,"* 157–72.

Katz, Esther, Peter C. Engelman, and Cathy Moran Hajo, eds. *The Selected Papers of Margaret Sanger*. Vol. 4, *'Round the World for Birth Control, 1920–1966*. Chicago: University of Illinois Press, 2016.

Kaufert, Patricia A., and John D. O'Neil. "Cooptation and Control: The Reconstruction of Inuit Birth." *Medical Anthropology Quarterly* 4, no. 4 (1990): 427–42.

Kevles, Daniel. *In the Name of Eugenics: Genetics and the Uses of Human Heredity*. Cambridge, MA: Harvard University Press, 1995.

Kline, Wendy. *Bodies of Knowledge: Sexuality, Reproduction, and Women's Health in the Second Wave*. Chicago: University of Chicago Press, 2010.

– *Building a Better Race: Gender, Sexuality, and Eugenics from the Turn of the Century to the Baby Boom*. Berkeley: University of California Press, 2001.

Kluchin, Rebecca. *Fit to be Tied: Sterilization and Reproductive Rights in America, 1950–1980*. New Brunswick, NJ: Rutgers University Press, 2011.

Ladd-Taylor, Molly. "Contraception or Eugenics? Sterilization and 'Mental Retardation' in the 1970s and 1980s." *Canadian Bulletin of Medical History* 31, no. 1 (2014): 189–212.

– *Fixing the Poor: Eugenic Sterilization and Child Welfare in the Twentieth Century*. Baltimore: Johns Hopkins University Press, 2017.

LaRocque, Emma. "Métis and Feminist: Ethical Reflections on Feminism, Human Rights and Decolonization." In Green, ed., *Making Space*, 53–71.

Lavell-Harvard, D. Memee, and Jeannette Corbiere Lavell. "Thunder Spirits: Reclaiming the Power of Our Grandmothers." In Lavell-Harvard and Corbiere Lavell, eds., *"Until Our Hearts are On the Ground,"* 1–12.

– eds. *"Until Our Hearts Are on the Ground": Aboriginal Mothering, Oppression, Resistance and Rebirth*. Toronto: Demeter Press, 2006.

Law Reform Commission of Canada. "Protection of Life: Sterilization: Implications for Mentally Retarded and Mentally Ill Persons." Working Paper No. 24. Ottawa, 1979.

Lawrence, Jane. "The Indian Health Service and the Sterilization of Native American Women." *American Indian Quarterly* 24, no. 3 (2000): 400–19.

Leavitt, Judith Walzer. *Brought to Bed: Childbirth in America, 1750–1950*. 1986; Oxford University Press, 1993.

"The Legal Aspects of Sterilization, reprint from the Ontario Medical Review." Editorial. *Alberta Medical Review* 14, no. 3 (1949): 53.

Leon, Sharon. *An Image of God: The Catholic Struggle with Eugenics.* Chicago: University of Chicago Press, 2013.

Lilar, Suzanne. *Le malentendu du deuxième sexe.* Paris: Université Presses du France, 1969.

Lišková, Kateřina. *Sexual Liberation, Socialist Style: Communist Czechoslovakia and the Science of Desire, 1945–1989.* Cambridge: Cambridge University Press, 2018.

Livingstone, E.S. "Vasectomy: A Review of 3200 Operations." *Canadian Medical Association Journal* 105, no. 10 (1971): 1065.

Lombardo, Paul A. *Three Generations, No Imbeciles: Eugenics, the Supreme Court, and Buck v. Bell.* Baltimore: Johns Hopkins University Press, 2008.

Lord, Alexandra M. *Condom Nation: The U.S. Government's Sex Education Campaign from World War I to the Internet.* Baltimore: Johns Hopkins University Press, 2010.

Luther, Emily. "Whose 'Distinctive Culture'? Aboriginal Feminism and R. v. Van der Peet." *Indigenous Law Journal* 8, no. 1 (2010): 27–53.

Lux, Maureen. *Separate Beds: A History of Indian Hospitals in Canada, 1920s–1980s.* Toronto: University of Toronto Press, 2016.

Magee, Kathryn. "'For Home and Country': Education, Activism, and Agency in Alberta Native Homemakers' Clubs, 1942–1970." *Native Studies Review* 18, no. 2 (2009): 27–49.

Malacrida, Claudia. *A Special Hell: Institutional Life in Alberta's Eugenic Years.* Toronto: University of Toronto Press, 2015.

"Male Sterilization: A Striking Change since *Maclean's* First Report" *Maclean's*, 15 December 1962.

Manuel, George, and Michael Posluns. *The Fourth World: An Indian Reality.* Don Mills, ON: Collier-Macmillan Canada, 1974.

Marcil-Gratton, Nicole, and Evelyne Lapierre-Adamcyk. "Sterilization in Quebec." *Family Planning Perspectives* 15, no. 2 (1983): 73–8.

Marsh, Margaret, and Wanda Ronner. *The Fertility Doctor: John Rock and the Reproductive Revolution.* Baltimore: Johns Hopkins University Press, 2008.

McCallum, Mary Jane. "This Last Frontier: Isolation and Aboriginal Health." *Canadian Bulletin of Medical History* 22, no. 1 (2005): 103–20.

McLaren, Angus. *Our Own Master Race: Eugenics in Canada, 1885–1945.* Toronto: McClelland & Stewart, 1990.

McLaren, Angus, and Arlene Tigar McLaren. *The Bedroom and the State: The Changing Practices of Contraception and Abortion in Canada, 1880–1997.* Toronto: Oxford University Press, 1997.

McTavish, Lianne. "Abortion in New Brunswick." *Acadiensis* 44, no. 2 (2015): 107–30.

Molyneaux, Heather. "Controlling Conception: Images of Women, Safety, Sexuality and the Pill in the Sixties." In *Gender, Health, and Popular Culture: Historical Perspectives*, ed. Cheryl Krasnick Warsh, 65–88. Waterloo: Wilfrid Laurier University Press, 2011.

Muir, Leilani. *A Whisper Past: Childless after Eugenic Sterilization in Alberta, A Memoir by Leilani Muir.* Victoria, BC: Friesen Press, 2014.

Murphy, Michelle. *The Economization of Life.* Durham: Duke University Press, 2017.

Norris, Mary Jane, and Stewart Clatworthy. "Urbanization and Migration Patterns of Aboriginal Populations in Canada: A Half Century in Review (1951 to 2006)." *Aboriginal Policy Studies* 1, no. 1 (2011): 13–77.

O'Brien, Gerald. *Framing the Moron: The Social Construction of Feeble-Mindedness in the American Eugenic Era.* Manchester: Manchester University Press, 2013.

O'Neil, John D. "Self-Determination, Medical Ideology and Health Services in Inuit Communities." In *Northern Communities: The Prospects for Empowerment*, ed. Gurston Dacks and Ken Coates, 33–50. Edmonton: Boreal Institute for Northern Studies, 1988.

"Ontario Sterilization Ban Extended in Order to Allow Discussion of Substitute Consent Issue." *Canadian Family Physician* 25 (November 1979): 1285, 1293.

Orr, Jackie. *Panic Diaries: A Genealogy of Panic Disorder.* Durham: Duke University Press, 2006.

Osennontion (Marlyn Kane) and Skonaganleh:rá. "Our World according to Osennontion and Skonaganleh:rá." *Canadian Woman Studies* 10, no. 2–3 (1989): 7–19.

Ouellette, Grace J.M.W. *The Fourth World: An Indigenous Perspective on Feminism and Aboriginal Women's Activism.* Halifax: Fernwood, 2002.

Owram, Doug. *Born at the Right Time: A History of the Baby Boom Generation.* Toronto: University of Toronto Press, 1996.

Palmer, Beth. "Abortion on Trial: Abortion Tribunals in the 1970s and 1980s." In Stettner, Burnett, and Hay, eds., *Abortion*, 114–32.

– "'Lonely, Tragic, but Legally Necessary Pilgrimages': Transnational Abortion Travel in the 1970s." *Canadian Historical Review* 92, no. 4 (2011): 637–64.

Palmer, Bryan D. *Canada's 1960s: The Ironies of Identity in a Rebellious Era.* Toronto: University of Toronto Press, 2009.

Parry, Manon. *Broadcasting Birth Control: Mass Media and Family Planning*. New Brunswick, NJ: Rutgers University Press, 2013.

Patton, Karissa. "'We Were Having Conversations That Weren't Comfortable for Anybody, but We Were Feisty': Re-conceiving Student Activism against Reproductive Oppression in Calgary and Lethbridge during the 1960s and 1970s." Honours thesis, University of Lethbridge, 2013.

Pauktuutit Inuit Women's Association. "Pauktuutit: Inuit Women's Association." Letter to the Premier of the Government of Nunavut. *Canadian Woman Studies*, 10, no. 2–3 (1989): 137–8.

Paul, Diane. *The Politics of Heredity: Essays on Eugenics, Biomedicine, and the Nature-Nurture Debate*. Albany: State University of New York Press, 1998.

Peters, Evelyn. "Aboriginal People in Urban Areas." In *Visions of the Heart: Canadian Aboriginal Issues*, ed. David Long and Olive Patricia Dickason, 237–70. Toronto: Nelson, 1998.

– "'Our City Indians': Negotiating the Meaning of First Nations Urbanization in Canada, 1945–1975." *Historical Geography* 30 (2002): 75–92.

Pichot, André. *The Pure Society: From Darwin to Hitler*. Translated by David Fernbach. London: Verso Books, 2009. Originally published as *La société pure: De Darwin à Hitler* (Paris: Flammarion, 2000).

Pile, John, and Mark Barone. "Demographics of Vasectomy – USA and International." *Urologic Clinics North America* 36, no. 3 (2009): 295–305.

Powell, Marion, and Raisa Deber. "Why Is the Number of Pregnancies among Teenagers Decreasing?" *Canadian Medical Association Journal* 127, no. 6 (1982): 493–5.

Primeau, Paul. "A Social History of the Eugenic Movement: The Enactment of the Sexual Sterilization Act S.A. 1928 and Its Effect on Indian and Metis People." Honours thesis, Lakehead University, 1998.

Rebick, Judy. *Ten Thousand Roses: The Making of a Feminist Revolution*. Toronto: Penguin, 2005.

Revie, Linda. "More Than Just Boots! The Eugenic and Commercial Concerns behind A.R. Kaufman's Birth Controlling Activities." *Canadian Bulletin of Medical History* 23, no. 1 (2006): 119–43.

Richards, Michael T. "Vasectomy … as an Office Procedure." *Canadian Medical Association Journal* 109, no. 5 (1973): 394, 386.

Rosenfeld, Joseph. *The Orgiastic Near East*. Canoga Park, CA: Viceroy Books, 1968.

Ross, Loretta. "What Is Reproductive Justice?" In *Reproductive Justice Briefing Book: A Primer on Reproductive Justice and Social Change*, n.d. [2007], 4–5. Accessed 3 September 2019. https://www.law.berkeley. edu/php-programs/courses/fileDL.php?fID=4051.

Roszak, Theodore. *The Making of a Counter Culture: Reflections on the Technocratic Society and Its Youthful Opposition*. Garden City, NY: Anchor Books, 1969.

Rutherford, Scott. "Canada's Other Red Scare: Rights, Decolonization, and Indigenous Political Protest in the Global Sixties." Ph.D. diss., Queen's University, 2011.

Ryan, Joan. *Wall of Words: The Betrayal of the Urban Indian*. Toronto: PMA Books, 1978.

Samson, Amy. "Eugenics in the Community: Gendered Professions and Eugenic Sterilization in Alberta, 1928–1972." *Canadian Bulletin of Medical History* 31, no.1 (2014): 143–63.

Schlesinger, Benjamin, ed. *Family Planning in Canada: A Source Book*. Toronto: University of Toronto Press, 1974.

Schoen, Johanna. *Choice and Coercion: Birth Control, Sterilization, and Abortion in Public Health and Welfare*. Chapel Hill: University of North Carolina Press, 2005.

Sethna, Christabelle. "All Aboard? Canadian Women's Abortion Tourism, 1960–1980." In *Gender, Health, and Popular Culture: Historical Perspectives*, ed. Cheryl Krasnick Warsh, 89–108. Waterloo: Wilfrid Laurier University Press, 2011.

Sethna, Christabelle, and Gayle Davis, eds. *Abortion across Borders: Transnational Travel and Access to Abortion Services*. Baltimore: Johns Hopkins University Press, 2019.

Sethna, Christabelle, and Steve Hewitt. "Clandestine Operations: The Vancouver Women's Caucus, the Abortion Caravan, and the RCMP." *Canadian Historical Review* 90, no. 3 (2009): 463–96.

– *Just Watch Us: RCMP Surveillance of the Women's Liberation Movement in Cold War Canada*. Montreal and Kingston: McGill-Queen's University Press, 2018.

Sethna, Christabelle, Beth Palmer, Katrina Ackerman, and Nancy Janovicek. "Choice, Interrupted: Travel and Inequality of Access to Abortion Services since the 1960s." *Labour/Le Travail* 71 (Spring 2013): 29–48.

Shiva, Mira, and Vandana Shiva. "Population and Environment: An Indian Perspective." *Women & Environments* 13, no. 3–4 (1993): 20–1.

Shorter, Edward. *A History of Women's Bodies*. New York, Basic Books, 1982.

Shropshire, Sarah. "What's a Guy to Do? Contraceptive Responsibility, Confronting Masculinity and the History of Vasectomy in Canada." *Canadian Bulletin of Medical History* 31, no. 2 (2014): 161–82.

Simmons, Harvey. *From Asylum to Welfare*. Downsview, ON: National Institute on Mental Retardation, 1982.

Simon Population Trust. *Vasectomy: Follow-Up of a Thousand Cases*. London: Garden City Press, 1969.

Smith, Linda Tuhiwai. *Decolonizing Methodologies: Research and Indigenous Peoples*. 2nd ed. London: Zed Books, 2012.

Snyder, Emily. "Indigenous Feminist Legal Theory." *Canadian Journal of Women and the Law* 26, no. 1 (2014): 365–401.

Solinger, Rickie. *Reproductive Politics: What Everyone Needs to Know*. Oxford: Oxford University Press, 2013.

Statistics Canada. *Therapeutic Abortions 1972*. Ottawa: Information Canada, 1973.

– *Therapeutic Abortions 1973*. Ottawa: Information Canada, 1974.

– *Therapeutic Abortions 1975*. Ottawa: Information Canada, 1977.

– *Therapeutic Abortions, 1976*. Ottawa: Information Canada, 1979.

– *Therapeutic Abortions, 1977: Advance Information*. Ottawa: Information Canada, 1978.

Statistics Canada. Health Statistics Division. *Selected Therapeutic Abortion Statistics, 1970–1991*. Ottawa: Information Canada, 1994.

Statistics Canada. Institutional Care Statistics Section. *Some Facts about Therapeutic Abortions in Canada, 1970–1982*. Ottawa: Information Canada, 1984.

St. Denis, Verna. "Feminism Is for Everybody: Indigenous Women, Feminism and Diversity." In Green, ed., *Making Space*, 33–52.

Stepan, Nancy Leys. *The Hour of Eugenics: Race, Gender and Nation in Latin America*. New York: Cornell University Press, 1992.

Stern, Alexandra Minna. *Eugenic Nation: Faults and Frontiers of Better Breeding in Modern America*. 2nd ed. Oakland: University of California Press, 2016.

– "From Legislation to Lived Experience: Eugenic Sterilization in California and Indiana, 1907–79." In *A Century of Eugenics in America: From the Indiana Experiment to the Human Genome Era*, ed. Paul A. Lombardo, 95–116. Bloomington: Indiana University Press, 2011.

Stettner, Shannon, ed. *Without Apology: Writings on Abortion in Canada*. Edmonton: Athabasca University Press, 2016.

Stettner, Shannon, Kristin Burnett, and Travis Hay, eds. *Abortion: History, Politics and Reproductive Justice after Morgentaler*. Vancouver: UBC Press, 2017.

Stevenson, Allyson. *Intimate Integration: A History of the Sixties Scoop and the Colonization of Indigenous Kinship*. Toronto: University of Toronto Press, 2020.

– "Intimate Integration: A Study of Aboriginal Transracial Adoption in Saskatchewan, 1944–1984." Ph.D. diss., University of Saskatchewan, 2015.

Stillwell, Devon. "Interpreting the Genetic Revolution: A History of Genetic Counselling in the United States, 1930–2000." Ph.D. diss., McMaster University, 2013.

Stote, Karen. *An Act of Genocide: Colonialism and the Sterilization of Aboriginal Women*. Halifax: Fernwood, 2015.

– "An Act of Genocide: Eugenics, Indian Policy, and the Sterilization of Aboriginal Women in Canada." Ph.D. diss., University of New Brunswick, 2012.

Suzack, Cheryl. "Indigenous Feminisms in Canada." *NORA – Nordic Journal of Feminist and Gender Research* 23, no. 4 (2015): 261–74.

Suzack, Cheryl, Shari M. Huhndorf, Jeanne Perreault, and Jean Barman, eds. *Indigenous Women and Feminism: Politics, Activism, Culture*. Vancouver: UBC Press, 2010.

Tomes, Nancy. "The Patient as a Policy Factor: A Historical Case Study of the Consumer/Survivor Movement in Mental Health." *Health Affairs* 25, no. 3 (2006): 720–9.

Tone, Andrea. *Devices and Desires: A History of Contraceptives in America*. New York: Hill & Wang, 2001.

Trudeau, Pierre. "Just Society," In *The Essential Trudeau*, edited by Ron Graham, 16–20. Toronto: McClelland & Stewart, 1998.

Turda, Marius, ed. *The History of East-Central European Eugenics, 1900–1945: Sources and Commentaries*. London: Bloomsbury, 2015.

Turpel, Mary Ellen (Aki-Kwe). "Patriarchy and Paternalism: The Legacy of the Canadian State for First Nations Women." *Canadian Journal of Women and the Law* 6, no. 1 (1993): 174–92.

Udel, Lisa. "Revision and Resistance: The Politics of Native Women's Motherwork." *Frontiers* 22, no. 2 (2001): 43–62.

"Vasectomy: How One Couple Ended the Fear of Dangerous Pregnancies." *Chatelaine*, May 1963.

Warsh, Cheryl Krasnick, ed. *Gender, Health, and Popular Culture: Historical Perspectives*. Waterloo: Wilfrid Laurier University Press, 2011.

Watkins, Elizabeth. *On the Pill: A Social History of Oral Contraceptives, 1950–1970*. Baltimore: Johns Hopkins University Press, 1998.

Weaver, Sally. *Making Canadian Indian Policy: The Hidden Agenda,
1968–70.* Toronto: University of Toronto Press, 1981.

Weindling, Paul. *Victims and Survivors of Nazi Human Experiments:
Science and Suffering in the Holocaust.* London: Bloomsbury, 2014.

Williams, Carol, with Don Gill. "Campus Campaigns against
Reproductive Autonomy: The Canadian Centre for Bioethical Reform
Campus Genocide Awareness Project as Propaganda for Fetal Rights."
ActiveHistory.ca, n.d. [2014]. Accessed 3 May 2018. http://activehistory.
ca/papers/paper-18/.

Wolfensberger, Wolf. *The Principle of Normalization in Human Services.*
Toronto: National Institute on Mental Retardation, 1972.

Wolfers, David, and Helen Wolfers. "Vasectomania." *Family Planning
Perspectives* 5, no. 4 (1973): 196–9.

Index